"As a specialist in human behavior, I need tools that work. And this is what Serge Augier's *Ba Zi* does! It gives impactful insights on people's drivers and inner tensions, which are easily used to initiate change. This book will provide you with invaluable information that will shed light on your personality like no other."

—Caroline Chéneau, Clinical Psychologist,
Coach and Intercultural Specialist

"Ba Zi is one of the powerful and secret arts of the Ba Men Da Xuan tradition. It allows us to better understand who we are, our strengths and weaknesses, our resources and aspirations, but also our potential and how we manage our relationships with others. A better understanding of these elements allows us to enjoy a smooth life and to increase our chances of success."

—Sébastien Nunes, Head of Innovation and
Fintech at a leading European bank

"Serge Augier's understanding of the Ba Zi is second to none. Not only does he make complex and profound knowledge accessible to everyone, he also gives a clear methodology on how to use Ba Zi to manage your everyday life. It really is a life-transforming book!"

—Arnaud Bouvet, Chief Marketing Officer
at Cubiks and Business Psychologist

T0299650

by the same author

Shen Gong and Nei Dan in Da Xuan
A Manual for Working with Mind, Emotion,
and Internal Energy
Serge Augier
With translations by Isis Augier
Foreword by Dr. Yang, Jwing-Ming
ISBN 978 1 84819 260 7
eISBN 978 0 85701 208 1

of related interest

**Heavenly Stems and Earthly Branches
—TianGan DiZhi**
The Heart of Chinese Wisdom Traditions
Master Zhongxian Wu and Dr Karin Taylor Wu
Foreword by Fei BingXun
ISBN 978 1 84819 151 8
eISBN 978 0 85701 158 9

**Heavenly Stems and Earthly Branches
—TianGan DiZhi**
The Keys to the Sublime
Card Set
Master Zhongxian Wu and Dr Karin Taylor Wu
ISBN 978 1 84819 150 1

BA ZI
THE FOUR PILLARS OF DESTINY

Understanding Character, Relationships
and Potential Through Chinese Astrology

Serge Augier

With editorial support from
Henning Cederkvist and Henrik Cederkvist

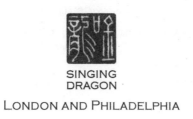

SINGING
DRAGON

LONDON AND PHILADELPHIA

First published in 2017
by Singing Dragon
an imprint of Jessica Kingsley Publishers
73 Collier Street
London N1 9BE, UK
and
400 Market Street, Suite 400
Philadelphia, PA 19106, USA

www.singingdragon.com

Library of Congress Cataloging in Publication Data
Names: Augier, Serge, author.
Title: Ba zi - the four pillars of destiny : understanding character,
    relationships and potential through Chinese astrology / Serge Augier.
Description: Philadelphia : Singing Dragon, 2016. | Includes index.
Identifiers: LCCN 2016004356 | ISBN 9781848192904 (alk. paper)
Subjects: LCSH: Astrology, Chinese. | Fortune-telling by birthdays--China
Classification: LCC BF1714.C5 A94 2016 | DDC 133.5/9251--dc23 LC
record available at http://lccn.loc.gov/2016004356

British Library Cataloguing in Publication Data
A CIP catalogue record for this book is available from the British Library

ISBN 978 1 84819 290 4
eISBN 978 0 85701 241 8

Printed and bound in Great Britain

Contents

CHAPTER 1

Introduction

He who knows others is learned;
He who knows himself is wise.

· *Lao Tzu, Dao De Jing*

The topic of this book is in the field of metaphysics, which is often hard to define, and from antiquity has changed and expanded to cover a wide range of subjects. Though the topic and knowledge contained in this book is not of Western origin but that of eastern philosophy, it is the universal understanding of Being, or "Being as such," which is the focus. The understanding of Man and his position in the universe goes beyond the mere physical manifestation.

Chinese metaphysics is a large and profound field of study, which encompasses much more than philosophical thinking and reflections. It is also a body of practical tools for very precise calculations and interpretations for understanding our Being and our interaction with the world. The most well-known of these is Feng Shui, which considers understanding how the environment and the surroundings affect us. It has very little to do with mirrors and plants positioned in the right spot of an apartment to make the energy of the home better! Although Feng Shui is not directly within the scope of this book, it will often be touched on because all the areas of Chinese metaphysics are interrelated. Nevertheless, these areas need to be addressed separately or we will get lost and confused. Chinese metaphysics enables us to understand the totality of a person's life and therefore can get quite complicated; but if we follow the structured steps and take our time and are patient, it can open up a whole new level of understanding of our own life.

The topic of this book, Ba Zi (Eight Characters), is far less well-known than Feng Shui, but is a very important part of understanding our Being. Here in the West most people have not heard of it, though we have most likely encountered it on a very superficial level. With every Chinese New Year we hear that it is the year of the rooster or the dragon, for example. And people who were born in these years have such and such a type of personality. This is a very broad generalization and does not hold much value. It is like reading the horoscope section in the newspaper and believing that what it says will actually happen to everybody who is a Gemini. And we know from our own experience that all the people we went to school with are not equal, even though we might have been born within the same Chinese year. Ba Zi goes far beyond these simple generalizations. It has been developed over countless generations and its depth is such that it could easily be studied at the level of a master's degree at a university today. However, from the basic principles of it we can get a lot of information that will help us in the pursuit of understanding our self.

> I went to the woods because I wished to live deliberately, to front only the essential facts of life, and see if I could not learn what it had to teach, and not, when I came to die, discover that I had not lived.

> *H.D. Thoreau*

Over recent years we have seen a rejuvenation in methods of self-discovery from age-old systems such as yoga, or modern variations of old practices such as mindfulness, in an attempt to understand ourselves better or as a reaction to the very hectic and dispersed life that we live. As we have gone from basic survival to living very comfortably in this modern age, we have time to reflect on our existence and the purpose of everything; but with this comfort can come overthinking. We are easily drawn away from being attentive to ourselves and slowing down, so people are realizing that we have to balance ourselves and understand ourselves better not from an external material perspective but from an internal observation. What we need to understand is that the traditional practices are like maps for the human being, a way to guide us towards our true nature, finding our meaning of life. The maps are there to help us to see and understand the different aspects of our personality (e.g. our talents and capacities) that are sometimes buried deep inside our mundane life. Learning what talent we possess helps us choose what we have to give to the world, the way we can interact with others. The deeper our understanding of who we are, the easier it is to achieve happiness and to do better in life.

> It is not only the most difficult thing to know oneself, but the most inconvenient one, too.
>
> *Josh Billings (H.W. Shaw)*

Ba Zi is applied psychology in that we seek to apply the theory to understanding both ourselves and others not just on a theoretical level but also practically. All the methods of Chinese metaphysics are meant to be used on a daily basis in our lives. With the eight characters, we seek to increase our ability to communicate and interact with other people in such a way that we can have a fruitful relationship with them. Again, we can draw from our own experiences of how we need to learn. Some people like studying by themselves, while others like to learn through group study. Some are more into examining things in depth and in detail, while others are content with only a superficial understanding. In understanding Ba Zi we can use it to convey what we need for the receiver of the information to understand it better. Again, if we for example knew the Ba Zi of a colleague who was difficult to interact with, then we could use it to understand them better in such a way that would make things easier not only for us but also for them. We need to emphasize that this is not about manipulation or control, but about understanding people better.

However, in the pursuit of knowledge of others, we need to take time to dig into our own self. Ba Zi will help us know our tendencies, what we are most likely to do in different aspects of our lives such as work and close personal relationships. As you can see, this is a large field, and we have to use it practically and look for the information that we need. With this knowledge of our self, we will move more towards the Daoist principle of non-resisting (Wu Wei), so that we do not resist ourselves. This means that we know when to act and when not to act because we understand the flow around us; we know the best timing for our actions.

> We are not permitted to choose the frame of our destiny. But what we put into it is ours.
>
> *D. Hammarskjöld*

The knowledge of who we are, of other people and of the world, is really what Daoist practice is about: Ba Zi is about trying to understand our destiny. The term "destiny" here is not the seemingly inevitable or necessary succession of events—that our life is already clearly set and that, whatever we do, the same things will happen. This is the Western or normal view of fate. Destiny in Daoism is about what potential we are given. It is not that we will have greatness if we do nothing, nor is it that everybody can achieve greatness with determination, positivity and some luck. It is about seeing what potential and limits we have, what we can actually achieve in life within our given frame.

This means that life is not fair in the view of a Daoist, but we work with what we have been given. Life for some will be easy, and we all know people who apparently glide through life on an unseemingly endless tide of luck, while others seem to be on an endless streak of bad luck. Just by looking to our close community or in the world in general, we see that life is not fair. Also, seemingly out of nowhere, people rise up to achieve greatness where others think there would be none. What potential we are given is what we are starting to study and understand in this book.

We know what we are but not what we may be.

Ophelia in Hamlet

Hence, with Ba Zi we can get a more in-depth view of what we can do and have to do to achieve our goals in life. These eight characters will show us the way to our own perfection, to the ideal image of ourselves. We will discover our talents and capacities, but also our weaknesses and our bad sides too. Consequently, the Ba Zi map gives us the possibility to develop our aptitudes and at the same time avoid our worst aspects. Additionally, Ba Zi can at some point be used with Feng Shui, both arts that can simplify our life by giving answers to our questions—and give directions to our everyday life.

Ba Zi is not easy, it's a lifelong process, but we can learn to use it at an introductory level—this is for all of us!

Ba Zi and its part in totality

Before we explore Ba Zi, we need to look at the Daoist view of Man in relation to the world and the universe. The Daoist view is of Man, heaven and earth being inseparable. Everything is joined and connected. While large outside forces affect the inner workings of Man, we must see that they view Man as a part of totality and not as something separate. While each of us is unique, we are all part of the world and the universe, making us also in a sense insignificant too. But the sum of all parts makes up the total. This view is not unique to Daoism but is a part of many spiritual traditions. The basis for Daoist practice is the understanding of Man or oneself in this totality. While understanding the uniqueness and insignificance at the same time, and being able to align oneself between heaven and earth, then Man can genuinely be happy. The image of this is Man standing between heaven and earth.

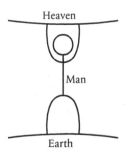

In this image, Man is holding the heavens while standing on the earth. This image is old and stems from the myth of the creation of the universe, with the mythical being Pan Gu who was born in an egg and pushed and separated it into heaven and earth. Heaven is pure spirit (yang) and earth is pure essence (yin), while Man is composed of both energies (yin and yang). This image explains the basis for understanding the Daoist view of Man in relationship to everything!

Yin and yang are core concepts in Daoism, and we will go into greater detail on these in later sections. We can think of yang as the most expansive and volatile, something we cannot grasp; and yin as the most concrete and material, something which is real.

With this image of Man as between heaven and earth, we can then look at the place of Ba Zi in the understanding of human nature. In order to do this, to understand better where Ba Zi fits into Chinese metaphysics, we need to look a little at what is called the three lucks (San Cai).

San Cai: the three lucks

Before we go into detail of the three lucks we will look at a short story that clarifies what one might consider luck:

> On the borders of the barbarian land lived a farmer with his family. It was a small farm and he only had one horse. One day his horse escaped and everyone in the village pitied him, but the farmer replied, "Why do you pity me? It might be a good thing!"
>
> A long time went by and his horse returned, accompanied by a majestic barbarian stallion. The people of the village were so happy for him, but the farmer replied, "Maybe it is a bad thing!"
>
> The farmer and his family enjoyed the help of the extra horse and his son loved to ride him. But one day he fell off the horse and was disabled! The village pitied him, and again the farmer replied, "What makes you think it is not a good thing?"
>
> One day the army of the land came and called all able-bodied men to arms because of the invading barbarian horde. Most of the young men of the village died, while the son of the farmer was spared because he was disabled.

From this story we see that, depending on the situation, something that seems good might turn out to be bad and something bad might turn out to be something good. As we gain more understanding of the study of Ba Zi we might see aspects of our self that we might consider bad, but in some instances in our life these so-to-say bad aspects of us might provide us with something good, and vice versa. In a simple example, consider that a person who is very good-hearted and likes to help people might meet a person who sees this and exploits this. Then this good trait is actually something that can be turned against us. It is valuable to keep this in mind when we start to delve deeper into Ba Zi so that we do not get stuck on our bad aspects or glorify our good sides, because they might change, depending on the situation.

We can now go into detail of the three lucks. They are Heaven luck, Man luck and Earth luck.

Heaven luck: Ba Zi

Heaven luck is what is given to us. We do not how or why, but it is our nature. It will comprise good aspects and bad aspects. It ranges from outward tendencies to deep unconscious behavior. Some people go through an easy life and others will struggle and have a hard time. It is not fair. This is Ba Zi, the heavenly mandate. There is not much we can change about it, but it is important that we understand it so that we can live life better.

Man luck: the practice

Man luck is what we actually can do for ourselves, a personal practice. The image describes the importance for Man to be in balance with himself, with himself and the earth, with himself and the heavens, and finally in balance between himself and heaven and earth. In other words, Man needs to be aligned between heaven and earth to correctly respond to the physical, energetic and mental aspects of any situation.

So what exactly do we mean by balance and alignment? Well, if we want to have a good life, we need to take care of our body, our vitality and our mind. We need to have the proper tools to work on ourselves. To work on the body we need Wai Gong (body), Nei Dan (energy) and Shen Gong (mind).

Wai Gong is physical exercises that are meant to give proper strength, rooting and structure. Nei Dan is the work of the breath and that which gives us vitality and energy in our daily life. Nei Dan constitutes all work on feeling the breath and getting in an intimate relation with our breath. Finally, to understand how our mind works and how actually we work, we need to work on the mind, Shen Gong. In Shen Gong, as we practice Nei Dan we start getting to know our mind and how it works.

With Wai Gong, Nei Dan and Shen Gong we can understand ourselves better in all aspects of our life. We will live more healthily and hence have more time for introspection and consequently a much better feeling of what is good or not good for us. Through understanding we can truly experience happiness.

When the body and mind are balanced, it is easier to understand other people as well, because a balanced human being is more relaxed and less influenced by emotions and ego. In addition, when aligned with heaven and earth, we will be able to adapt and exchange better with the world. In short, the first thing we need to understand from the image is that we need to practice and we need to take care of ourselves.

Earth luck: Feng Shui

Feng Shui is the third luck and is about how the environment and natural surroundings affect us. It is about how we organize the environment around us so that we align it with our Heaven luck and Man luck, making them optimal. While Heaven luck is what is given to us and, as we have said, there is not so much we can do with it, Earth luck is something we can do a lot to change.

This means that at some point in the study of Ba Zi it is joined with Feng Shui, giving us all we need to situate ourselves in time and space. Some people's actions will sometimes be very dependent on timing, while others can do mostly what they want when they want, but this is not within the scope of this book.

Before going further...

We can see the three lucks as a road trip where Heaven luck is the vehicle you have (car, bicycle, etc.) during your travels. The road is the Earth luck (highway or dirt road), and finally, the driver, which is us, is Man luck. So based upon the vehicle and the driver we have many options for traveling the road. It is important to understand that if the driver is a practitioner of the Way he should learn everything about driving (the car, the road, etc.) to make the road trip as pleasant as possible.

This is a short, but nevertheless important, introduction of the Daoist image of Man. To understand Ba Zi we need to understand how everything is connected in Daoist practice and its tools. If one wants to dig deep into the understanding of the human mind, it is very important to understand that not much comes out of such a study if one is not willing to start with oneself first, before trying to understand others. That is why Ba Zi is such a great tool. We can use it on ourselves to understand ourselves better with ourselves, but also ourselves with other people.

Finally, the image talks about Ba Zi and how important it is to understand and use it in relation with human beings. Through Ba Zi we get a much deeper understanding of the fundamental laws that lie behind every variant of personas that exist. It is the Daoist's system for applied psychology.

The origin of yin and yang
How did the theory start?
Daoism has a very long and rich history stretching back to the old shamanic traditions. From Native Americans to the Sami of the northern countries, the understanding of nature and Man's role in it has been central, as we have seen earlier in the description of Man between heaven and earth.

During the Yin Dynasty (c.1400–1100 BC) the Shaman Wu developed a system of interrogation of nature through a patient observation of the forces of nature. Through this careful study over generations, a view of the world and the universe developed whereby everything in the universe is constantly moving and changing—from night to day, from winter to summer, and so on; these gave way to the theory of yin and yang. The oldest written records of yin and yang are probably those which appear in the *Book of Changes* (the *Yi Jing*), whose first tablets were made around 700 BC. The system and theory was put in writing only towards 200 BC and comprised 64 hexagrams that explained all phenomena existing in nature. From the rise and fall of nations to the internal workings of Man, it is a complete theory of understanding changes in nature.

The *Yi Jing*

It is not possible to talk about Chinese metaphysics without saying something about the *Yi Jing*. This book is one of the oldest known Chinese texts of philosophy and divination. Along with the *Dao De Jing*, the *Yi Jing* is the most well-known classical Chinese work of ageless wisdom. Though it is mostly famous for divination, the *Yi Jing* is a lot more than that. Conveying the rhythms and laws of universe in a specific structure of 64 hexagrams, this ancient text opens the door to a deep understanding of our actions and the inevitable nature of change.

The Tao gives birth to one
one gives birth to two
two gives birth to three
three gives birth to ten thousand things
ten thousand things with yin at their backs
and yang in their embrace
and breath between for harmony

Dao De Jing, verse 42 (tr. Bill Porter)

In the figure below, we see the development of yin and yang from Tai Ji until the eight trigrams of heaven, lake, fire, thunder, wind, water, mountain and earth.

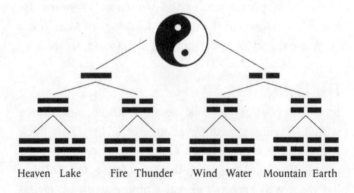

Heaven Lake   Fire Thunder   Wind Water   Mountain Earth

The 64 hexagrams are the 8×8 combinations of the trigrams. The four base hexagrams of the *Yi Jing* can be seen in the next figure.

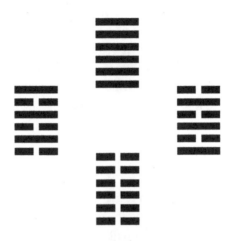

These four are the nucleus for the remaining 60 and give us the base for all situations. As previously mentioned in the above extract from the *Dao De Jing*, they describe everything, or the ten thousand things. If we look back at the image of Man between heaven and earth, this is the complete theory, with Ba Zi and Feng Shui arising from this. But know that the knowledge contained in the book is deep and can take a lifetime to master. The difficulty lies in the understanding of each hexagram, because very often the information and explanation is just one example of its interpretation. Each of the hexagrams should be adaptable to any situation that we might want to look at—from work and money to relationships, amongst many other things. So, from these 64 things, we should be able to explain everything.

Now that we have seen how things are connected, we must understand that this is just a brief overview. When it comes to Feng Shui and the *Yi Jing*, these need to be handled separately. Next we go into the details of yin and yang and five-element theory (Wu Xing), which together form the foundation of Ba Zi and all of Chinese metaphysics!

Yin and yang in detail

> Nothing that is can pause or stay;
> The moon will wax, the moon will wane,
> The mist and cloud will turn to rain,
> The rain to mist and cloud again,
> Tomorrow be today.

> *Henry Wadsworth Longfellow*

In nature, yin and yang are the existing opposites of any given phenomenon. Every phenomenon is composed of two polarities that appear in a relation of coherency. Yin and yang are in fact a generalization of the opposite aspects that appear in things, the phenomena bound by mutual relations. The one cannot exist without the other— for example, beautiful vs ugly, cold vs hot, dark vs light. Moreover, they are relative and not absolute. We cannot say that something is yin or yang without comparing it to something else. And, likewise, something that was defined as yang can again be divided into yin and yang. It is infinite!

This concept can apply as things or phenomena of opposed natures, but also as two opposite aspects of the same thing or the same phenomenon. The theory explains that the shape and function of the phenomenon are defined by the variance of the two different polarities. And it also says that no phenomenon persists eternally in its own nature. For example, the body responds to the environment unceasingly to find a relative balance that will reinstate either health or disease. Another example is of course the seasons. Each season is an endless number of phases within itself but also between the different seasons. When a season has begun, it is already transforming into something. No season ever actually starts or ends per se; rather, it transmutes into a new version of itself.

Each phenomenon, condition, position and state is endlessly undergoing change to retain balance of its yin and yang. They are not fixed, locked or constant but change mutually; for example, they are transmutations. These changes do not occur at random but at certain stages of evolution, regulated by nature.

Another way of explaining yin and yang is to look at three superimposed objects in relation to each other. The top object will then be yang and the bottom object will be yin, while the middle will be composed of yin and yang. We see this image also in the traditions where Man (yin and yang) stands between heaven (yang) and earth (yin), as described earlier.

> Life is a series of natural and spontaneous changes. Do not resist them; that only creates sorrow. Let reality be reality. Let things flow naturally forward in whatever way they like.
>
> *Lao Tzu*

On the basis of yin and yang theory, one can comprehend any phenomenon, according to the context, by defining what the yin is and what the yang is. Importantly, it is necessary to keep in mind the dynamic of interchange more than the definition of yin and yang and to manage to put into perspective the two concepts.

The four laws of yin and yang

Yin and yang theory dictates that these polarities have four different properties:

1. Opposites

2. Interdependence

3. Balance

4. Transformation.

OPPOSITES

This first law is most likely the one which people associate with their understanding of yin and yang—that yin and yang are opposites.

Each coexists to control the other, and through their opposition they maintain the dynamic balance needed for a certain phenomenon, thing or situation to exist. It is dynamic and provides the foundation for change in nature. To understand the duality of the world we must understand yin and yang. For there to be good there must be bad; when something is right then the opposite is wrong. This is the duality.

Yin	Yang
Darkness	Light
Moon	Sun
Sink	Rise
Shade	Brightness
Slow	Fast
Sunset	Sunrise
North	South
Earth	Heaven
Right	Left
Blood	Spirit
Matter	Energy
Structure	Function

INTERDEPENDENCE

Yin and yang cannot exist without the other. Each polarity has its own energy, forces and dynamics that the other is dependent upon to exist individually.

In traditional Chinese medicine it is as though each organ needs a structure in order to have a function. The structure is yin, while the function is yang; for example, the heart could not pump blood through the body if it was not constructed as it is. We see this also in the transportation of electricity: power lines give the structure and are yin, while energy is yang. There are numerous other examples: one is that a car could not transport us (yang) somewhere without an engine and wheels (yin). One thing to note regarding our understanding of yin and yang is that yin is structure and yang is function.

BALANCE

When one of the polarities shrinks, the other needs to grow, and vice versa. This is to keep the phenomenon existing within its given limits. It is like a mathematical equation such as $x+y=1$. The variables x and y can be anything as long as they sum to one. It is the same as when you spend money to buy something. By paying for something (decrease), you gain something else (increase).

From a Ba Zi standpoint, we will, for example, be looking at the balance of yin and yang. Too much yin or yang will often indicate a need for more balance. And in Chinese medicine, an excess of yin or yang will lead to disease.

TRANSFORMATION

When yang becomes too much it will change into its opposite, yin. If yin becomes too much it will change into yang. This means that both polarities can create the other. However, for the transformation to occur, the conditions need to be right and the timing needs to be correct. Things always fluctuate with varied amplitude, and it is only when optimal amplitude is timed with the correct conditions that a transformation is possible. For example, as a season reaches its peak, it consequently starts to change into its opposite; summer becomes winter.

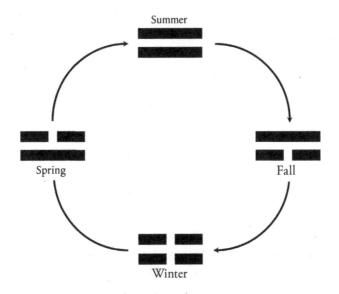

We see that summer is absolute yang and therefore is at its maximum. Then the lower line changes to yin and we are in fall. As the last yang rises, it gives way to a final yin that gives us winter. Winter is the absolute of yin and therefore must change. Moreover, when we get to spring, yang starts to rise and we return to summer; the cycle repeats itself.

This change from yin to yang or vice versa can be seen when training to develop one's strength and more muscles. You train and train—yang action—and when you have trained long enough (amplitude) and taken into account the correct diet and rest (conditions), you pass a threshold and obtain more muscles (yin); that is, yang action has produced more yin.

From this, we can see that yin and yang theory is the foundation that makes it possible to know and explain the world.

Wu Xing: the five elements

To understand Ba Zi we have to have a basic understanding not only of yin and yang, but also of the theory of the five elements (Wu Xing). Wu Xing can also be translated as five movements, phases or dynamics. This just simply restates that the five elements are not fixed conditions, but are *always* changing due to the natural evolution of things or in response to being forced in another direction. To simplify the concept we will use the five elements from now on, but remember that the elements are based upon yin/yang theory and hence always change relative to each other in order to maintain balance from either internal or external forces, or even an interplay between external and internal forces. That is why Wu Xing is also called the five phases, movements or dynamics.

The five elements are:

- wood (Mu)
- fire (Huo)
- earth (Tu)
- metal (Jin)
- water (Shui).

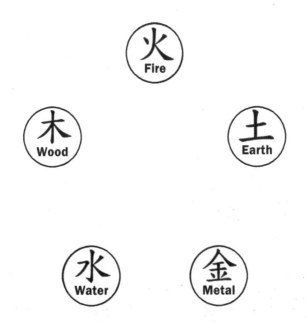

Compared with the theory of yin and yang, Wu Xing was invented rather more recently (300 BC). It was developed to rationalize and systemize the connection that could exist between different aspects in accordance with their properties, movements and interactions, like the theory of yin and yang. However, in contrast to yin/yang theory, which points to an infinite description of a phenomenon, Wu Xing was never meant to be rigidly accurate, but rather a general objective description of natural phenomena. Hence, five elements theory can only be understood by observing one element in relationship with the others. All Chinese metaphysics, for example Ba Zi and Feng Shui, uses Wu Xing to describe situations and relations to other people, places, circumstances, personalities and so on.

Interestingly, Wu Xing has been adopted by traditional Chinese medicine (TCM). In TCM, the theory of Wu Xing has been implemented by relating each of the five energetic organs—Liver, Spleen/Stomach, Kidney, Heart and Lungs—to a certain element: Liver is wood, Spleen/Stomach is earth, Kidney is water, Heart is fire and Lungs are metal. By placing each organ in relation to the Wu Xing it is possible to determine the physiological and pathological dynamics that exist in a patient, with each element generating another, controlling another and even being controlled by another.

Before we start to look more closely at Wu Xing we will provide an introduction to the different elements and their properties and examples of personality traits that these elements represent in Ba Zi. We will then describe the five cycles of Wu Xing and how Ba Zi uses this theory for understanding the relationship between people.

Wood

Wood is the expansive force that goes in all directions and towards the outside. It is not a finely directed energy like a laser beam, but more like light being deflected in all directions when it hits a reflective surface. It always wants to grow and expand and it needs freedom/space. That is why the image of a huge tree with its trunk, branches and roots is such a good example. The tree can only achieve this size if it has been given the space and time to develop. As the tree, the element of wood embodies the properties of stability, flexibility (but limited at the same time), growth and free expansion. In many ways the energy of wood is very similar to the expanding nature of fire.

Since the energy of wood is always expanding in all directions, it makes it difficult for this energy to be centered and focused on one thing.

The element of wood embodies knowledge. Knowledge is something that has taken time to seek and acquire, just as it takes time for a tree to grow. The branches of the tree reach out in all directions to cover an area as large as needed to get as much sunlight as needed to sustain the ever-growing trunk that is its core. The trunk is the growing knowledge that is fed by the branches.

In wood we also have intelligence, intuition and the development of the potential of the individual. To have strong intuition you need a sound level of knowledge. These properties are the yin and yang elements in the energy of wood.

Similar to the tree from the start of its development, there is already a defined potential. This means that as long as the tree is given its space and nutrients it will grow into whatever it was supposed to become. This is the energy of wood, the potential of becoming whatever it is supposed to grow into under the right circumstances. We can see this also in children when they grow up. The right upbringing and education give the child the possibility of evolving into what is deep inside of them.

All this expanding energy is strongly associated with creativity and the expression of oneself. The potential of what is inside needs to come out and blossom.

The element of wood represents the Liver in TCM and it is an essential part of the mind (Hun) for managing emotions. The function of the Liver is to make the qi flow smoothly in the body. So when the Liver energy or wood energy is stagnating or being obstructed, people get frustrated and agitated—the expanding wood energy is being stopped from growing, and hence friction occurs.

Finally, water produces wood, and wood produces fire.

A WOOD PERSON

A wood person is straight and clear in their way and thus very honest. As the tree they need stability and to stay in one place. Being the tall tree, they easily get a good overview of things and thus are good at seeing the bigger picture.

The expansive energy of wood makes these people easily frustrated if things are in their way or if things are not going fast enough. They also have a tendency to want to be recognized, since they are the tallest tree and everyone should look up to them. They need to have a direction or they will get confused.

Fire

Fire is the ascending movement. That is, fire is the energy/ movement that is *always* rising towards the sky, top or peak. Its momentum is constantly upwards to go beyond wherever it started. It has to reach new heights all the time or it will weaken. It is like making a camp fire. From the first spark that has ignited the wood the fire will always continue to burn and stretch itself from the wood as long as it has fuel to burn. But you will also see that putting something on top of the camp fire will quell the fire or even quench it if there is too much on top.

The fire therefore needs space to expand/ascend and it also continuously needs to be fueled or it will eventually consume itself.

Fire is also what cleanses and makes things possible to come back from the ashes/be reborn. For example, after a blazing forest fire, everything has been burned to the ground, but from all that ash plants grow back, and even new plants that were not existing there before are given a possibility to take root and grow there. Even the animals and insects come back, taking up their residences and prospering. Fire can make old things go away and enable new things to enter.

This also means that fire is the element that brings heat, light, life and illumination. Fire replaces the darkness with light and brings forth that which was not seen. Fire is what rises to the sky and, hence, gets a good perspective of the earth, while being able to shine upon everything that is below.

Fire is of course also the sun! It is the center of attention in the blue sky while it is shining down upon the earth with all its intensity and power. There is nothing more captivating in the sky than the sun. And even during cloudy days the heat from the sun will eventually burn through and again cast its light upon what lies below. The sun is also something we can use as a compass. We know that it rises in the east in the morning and descends in the west in the evening, and at noon it points us towards the south. Of course it is a bit more complicated than that, but in short the sun always gives us a direction and lights up the path to go there.

Even during the night the sun is indirectly showing us the way by shining upon the moon. If the moon rises before the sun has set, the illuminated side will be the west. If the moon rises after midnight, the illuminated side will be the east. This obvious discovery provides us with a rough east–west reference during the night using the moon that is directly under the control of the sun. You can say that the moon is the yin of the sun. The sun is always present in its entirety.

In the context of light, fire also promotes communication, ideas and social interaction. Illumination is the symbol of awakening, quickening and understanding. From fire the light is produced, and from the light everything that was difficult to discern since it was obscured by the shadows is revealed. When things are obvious it is easier to approach and sociably interact. It is so much easier to understand a topic when things are made clear; and when it is clear you can build upon this understanding and create something new from what is already there. Ideas can come so much more easily when we see things clearly.

Fire is the Heart, and hence fire reaches out to connect people, making it possible to open conversation and communication.

Fire is created from wood and produces earth. In the process of consuming, it also produces something, that is, it leaves something behind that has the capacity to be a source for something new.

Since fire is linked to the Heart in TCM we also find everything concerning love, joy, unity, the spirit (Shen), conscience and inspiration in the element of fire. The capacity to enjoy life and to know what makes one happy lies in fire. As long as the fire is burning strongly enough, the light can illuminate all dark corners and consequently make all possibilities visible. It is like hiking in the dark. If you have low light conditions it is very difficult to see any further than your feet sometimes, but as soon as you turn on your torch the whole landscape opens up to you and you can take the right route based upon what you want and need to do. You can even go into detail of how you want to organize the rest of the trip based upon this "little" step of lighting up the terrain.

The ideogram for fire is a central flame and two sparks.

A FIRE PERSON

In general, a fire person is warm, passionate and loving. As explained earlier, the rising and ascending flame makes it impossible for a fire person not to want to be the center of attention. It is impossible for him/her not to be seen. A fire person has an innate need to be noticed or the fire will be quelled, as in the camp fire analogy. Actually, being recognized is more inclined to happen to a fire person because they will always rise higher than anyone else. They will always be the innovator and communicator that demands attention. Their captivating personality is mainly due to their radiant appearance, but also because they are excellent communicators. They have the capacity to make things clear (illuminating the situation). People easily recognize them since they have the tendency to be very outspoken and loud. Also, fire people always want to help people by telling them what they feel is right.

They can easily become loners if they don't take care since they are always going towards new things (the continuous ascending movement). This means that in relationships they have a tendency to want to move on to another when they see something new that they want to get, achieve or apprehend. It is not that they do not have the capacity to love; on the contrary, they are very passionate and caring—it is just that when they see something better or see something wrong, they have the tendency to go towards the new.

Since fire always consumes its source, a fire person will deplete themselves of energy very easily. The fire person needs continual replenishment of the fuel they have burned away; just as when the fuel tank is empty, the car will no longer drive! They need to take care not to do too much or eventually they will hit the wall and suffer burn-out. The trick for a fire person is to have the optimum camp fire that can keep them warm and make the food they need, while at the same time not consuming too much wood. It is energy economics in real life!

Earth

The element of earth is the movement that stabilizes and goes from outward to inward. Earth is movement/phase/energy that goes inwards and condenses. It is the element that makes it possible to sow and harvest. Earth represents the intellectual work to consequently do or get something later. The energy of earth is the capacity to plan and discern what is needed.

For example, you live in a secluded area and you need to be able to take care of yourself. What do you do? Well, you start to consider all the options you have, and what is really important to have (food, communication) and what is not so important (access to a soda machine). This is part of earth, to rationalize and discern, and to make the right choices—if you want corn, you plant corn seeds and not potatoes. If you want a healthy body, you eat (sow) a well-balanced diet to balance out what your body needs (harvest). If you want a successful business, you put in the effort of building a good foundation for your business.

As in nature, earth represents production and transformation. For example, in the deepest parts of the earth we find riches that have been transformed over millennia from simple minerals/elements to valuable diamonds and other gems. This is the property of the earth to transform things. And remember the quality of what you have—or put in the earth—determines what it can be transformed into. If you want good wine you need to sow seeds from good grapes or else the wine will not become good. It is that simple.

Earth also represents the qualities of rooting and having a practical spirit. The earth condenses and keeps you grounded and sound like the base of a building. Earth is like a mountain: it stands there immovable and towering. The mountain is unyielding and will even stand the test of time. This is the energy of earth. It concretizes things, making them more clear and understandable. It is the logic of things and not creativity or phantasm. Hence, that which is logic can consequently become a practical thing. Earth is everything that is represented in all the laws and principles that you can find in science, engineering, mechanics and so on. Again, it is easy to see that earth is the base and foundation for making something and seeing things clearly for what they are. This ability to analyze and to make critical judgments is a part of earth. Earth lies in the art of contemplation and hence in the Yi part of the mind.

The organ for this element in TCM is the Spleen/Stomach. So when the Spleen/Stomach functions well, you have a clear mind and it is easy to understand/comprehend things. By contrast, too much earth energy brings indifference, laziness and casualness. Remember that the image of earth is also the mountain. The mountain does not have a tendency to move. The mountain is the epitome of stillness. So too much earth also signifies that there is too much mental regurgitation/activity/repeating thoughts, and this consequently very often leads to anxiety and worrying.

AN EARTH PERSON

Now, as the mountain, earth people are quiet and resilient people. They will endure hardship without complaint and they just wait for things to pass by. On the other hand, they will have difficulty responding quickly to situations. They are generally a bit slow on the trigger. The situation will come over them and then they will act. They will plan things and think a bit too much before deciding what to do. They will know what to do, but fast decision making is not their thing. If it seems like they are reacting quickly it just means that they already have thought about it for a long time. Being earth means being slow, but at the same time they find their center very easily. It is like a well-anchored ship. The ship will stay where it is since it has been properly secured to the bottom. Therefore, being earth makes you a very stable and strong-willed person, but also quite egotistical at the same time.

As the soil that can absorb a lot of water, it also has a certain capacity before the ground cannot take any more. The amount of water after a while starts to dissolve and move the earth. This image explains how earth people digest emotions and thoughts. They have difficulties handling their own and others' emotions and consequently are easily prone to worries and anxiety. And finally, as the mountain or earth, they prefer to stay still and consequently need to ensure they have movement in their life or they can become very lazy.

Metal

The element of metal represents that which is malleable and hard at the same time. It is what produces water and as such has the capacity to be malleable and strong. Metal is what gathers, collects, cuts and slices. Metal is justice and righteousness. Metal defines the distinction between two sources—right and wrong, left and right or up and down. For example, the energy of metal is what sets the boundaries of things—what should be there or not. In a social aspect it is what defines the boundaries between countries, communities, counties, neighbors and so on.

Metal defines the differences between cultures, people and social settings. It defines what is socially acceptable. It tells you what values lie within a person, a group, a country and the world, relative to each other. Everything that defines human interrelationships is part of the energy of metal.

Metal represents the wisdom and capacity to see the truth and face up to it—for example, what is good for us, and what is not. As metal, it defines a form of rigidity that has difficulty seeing the more subtle and detailed parts of things. It cannot distinguish the finer things where differences between right and wrong, high and low or yes or no have a very fine line or lie in the gray area. Metal is generally very black-and-white.

Metal has the quality to restore the essence but also to restrict. In addition, metal is hard and resists things easily. It will take a large amount of force to break metal, but over time it can wither due to corrosion and rust. It needs to be taken care of or it will eventually lose its strength.

A very important aspect of metal is that it reflects light—whatever you shine on it will reflect the same back. It is therefore important to take care of metal and keep it shiny, so whatever you shine upon it will be reflected back with at least the same strength and purity. If you want metal to discern and separate things correctly, it needs to be properly sharp so that it does not cut imprecisely and clumsily. If you want the butcher to cut your meat correctly and even be able to trim and clean the meat, he will need a good, strong and sharp blade.

Regarding the organs in TCM, metal represents the Lungs (Po), and hence it is associated with the breath, body energy and the ability to condense and emit. Strong Lungs give strong qi and consequently strong health. If the Lungs are weakened (e.g. the metal blade becomes dull), you will consequently suffer from fatigue and have difficulties digesting emotions. The quality of the Lungs defines the quality of the metal blade to work properly.

A METAL PERSON

People of the element of metal are known to be altruistic and care for other people. They are tough and have a strong sense of justice. It is very easy for them to cut through situations and tell people exactly how things should be or how they are. But since their view is very much black-and-white, they are not always the best diplomats when there needs to be a bit more subtlety in communication. Metal people are excellent soldiers due to their hardness and ability to handle life-and-death situations.

Additionally, metal people need to be careful regarding their behavior. They can very easily become too hard and non-forgiving, so they need to tame themselves. They easily forget that metal can also be malleable, but of course metal is never like water. Finally, metal people have a tendency to think too much and hence be susceptible to worries.

Water

The element of water defines everything that is fluid, in constant change and moving. Like a river it will always find a way to travel through terrain and always have momentum. Water needs to circulate/move or, like a pool that has nowhere to go, will become stagnant and filled with algae and sediment. The energy of water needs to move or it will become polluted. Water is also the source of life in nature. Even the driest desert will come to life after a rainfall. Water is the basis for all life and it nourishes the earth. But equally, as important as it is for sustaining life, it is also capable of destroying it. If too much water moves, then floods occur, the dam breaks or a huge tsunami will hit the shore.

These properties of water are the primal source for adaptation in life. It has the capacity to change in any given situation; but within movement lies the fear of stopping, and hence the energy of water is limited by fear. Therefore, we say that stagnant water is the source of disease, confusion or hindrance in life. Things need to always move or they are dead, as in yin/yang theory. The ideogram is the current of water.

As a force, water is descending (to the bottom) like a waterfall or like a river coming down from the mountains. In water lies the energetic potential of doing things or creating things. Water is the underlying potential to make things come to life. It is the source of life and is directly coupled to sexual energy and to procreation.

Water preserves energy, knowledge, wisdom and secrets in the depth of its form. But to get access to these treasures the water needs to be calm. If you are looking for a shipwreck in a turbulent sea you will have difficulty locating it between all the powerful movements on the surface and the huge difficulties of seeing through the water that has stirred up all the particles from the sea bottom. It is only in a tranquil lake or sea that you will be able to see things properly/clearly.

Water is also the energy executed by the will to reach its aims. Water is the capacity to act and do, and the only thing that hinders it from acting is fear. In water we also find introspection, insightfulness, self-assurance and internal force.

The water element represents the Kidneys in TCM, the force of will to take action and the ability to survive (Zhi). It is in the Kidneys that your life essence is contained, but also all of your potential in life. Your life force and your heritage lie in the Kidneys. So if your Kidneys start to fail it actually touches all of the other energetic organs as described in TCM, just as in nature when life does not flourish if there is little clean water. The absence of water affects everything, and this is also described in the TCM for the Kidneys, as represented by the water element. Metal creates water, and water creates and nourishes wood.

A WATER PERSON

A water person is considered wise and intuitive and able to understand people on a deep level. They easily adapt to new situations and circumstances, but as water they always move to prevent themselves from stagnating. Consequently they need to take care so that they do not lose their perspective on things. Being the element that contains knowledge, they are excellent at teaching people and touching them.

As this element, they need to stay in motion or they will not be happy. They also need to stay focused because they are easily dispersed and not very centered; water always wants to move and not stay at the same place for too long. Like the river running down a valley, water will turn and bend at any obstacle or sometimes just run through the hindrance if it can. The river very seldom runs straight.

Reinforcing is another important part: The relationship between the elements

> The meeting of two personalities is like the contact of two chemical substances: if there is any reaction, both are transformed.
>
> *C.G. Jung*

As mentioned above, Wu Xing explains the five elements and their possible interaction patterns or cycles. There are four different cycles in Wu Xing and we need to understand them to be able to interpret Ba Zi. Generally speaking, Ba Zi takes into account that all people portray a certain type of persona that can be explained by one of the elements. And these different personas interact differently with each other, depending upon which elements they are. For example, a fire person interacts differently with an earth person than they do with a water person.

The Wu Xing cycles describe how things normally should flow (creation cycle), go against what is normally situated (insulting cycle), dominate over certain aspects (controlling cycle), and finally how one element can drain another (exhausting cycle). Reinforcing is another important part.

1. *The creation cycle (Xiang Sheng)*. Wood creates fire, fire creates earth, earth creates metal, metal creates water, and water creates wood.

2. *The insulting cycle (Xiang Wu)*. Earth insults wood, wood insults metal, metal insults fire, fire insults water, and water insults earth.

3. *The controlling cycle (Xiang Ke)*. Wood controls earth, earth controls water, water controls fire, fire controls metal, and metal controls wood.

4. *The exhausting cycle (Xiang Cheng)*. Fire exhausts wood, wood exhausts water, water exhausts metal, metal exhausts earth, and earth exhausts fire.

5. *Reinforcing.* The same element reinforces the same element. For example, if you have two fires it is reinforced in Ba Zi, but if you have six fires it is too much.

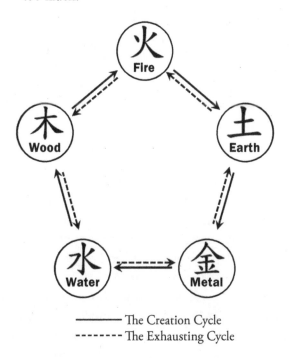

——— The Creation Cycle
- - - - - - The Exhausting Cycle

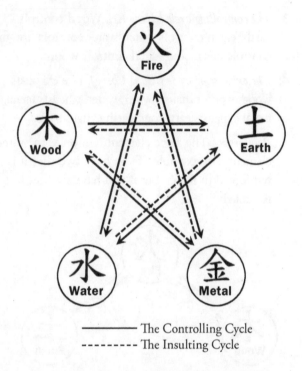

——————— The Controlling Cycle
- - - - - - - - - The Insulting Cycle

Now that we have introduced the different cycles we can start to understand how different personas interact with each other depending upon which element they are. Let us choose the example of a fire person interacting with different kinds of people and see how that fire person responds to the different situations.

The natural cycle of things is what we can observe in the creation cycle. Every element is produced from another element. Or, explained in another way, every element is nourished by another element. So in this context we see that a fire person is nourished by the interaction with a wood person, since wood creates fire. We can also see that what is nourishing the other is also exhausted by doing so: for example, wood creates fire (creation cycle); fire exhausts wood (exhausting cycle).

From the controlling cycle the fire person would be dominated and controlled by a water person. This may sound a bit negative but it actually is not. Being under control means that there is one that is yin and the other that is yang—a natural coexisting partnership.

The opposite of the controlling cycle is the insulting cycle. Here we have a fire person that is too strong for the water person to handle, and in this case things are not in balance or natural.

Wu Xing and yin/yang

Though we will not yet go into detail on this topic, it is important here to have some understanding of how Wu Xing and yin/yang interact together. In the theory of yin and yang we stated that yin and yang are opposites, so for everything there is a polarity. So too for the elements. These are also referred to in Ba Zi as the Tian Gan (Heavenly Stems). For now we will just give a brief summary of the ten different combinations (see the next table).

These Tian Gan will then have their own variations of the elements with their strengths and weaknesses. It is good to think a little about these images and what they actually mean in relation to a person and their behavior because they will enable a better understanding of Ba Zi later on.

Element	Polarity	Chinese name	Image
Wood	Yang	Jia	A huge tree
	Yin	Yi	Bamboo
Fire	Yang	Bing	The sun
	Yin	Ding	A candle
Earth	Yang	Wu	A mountain
	Yin	Ji	A candle
Metal	Yang	Geng	An axe
	Yin	Xin	Jewelry
Water	Yang	Ren	Tsunami
	Yin	Gui	Mist

What is Ba Zi?

Up to now we have discussed several aspects of the Daoist view of Man, but also which tools are primarily applied in a Daoist practice. As mentioned earlier, the basic concepts of yin and yang and the five elements are essential theories for understanding Ba Zi.

We will now give a short overview of Ba Zi and how a chart actually looks on paper.

Ba Zi is a tool that was developed to understand the different psychological traits of Man, and for this purpose the traditions applied their knowledge of yin and yang and the elements to a whole new context. They saw that each person has one major characteristic trait that is given by one of the five elements (the Wu Xing), and is called the Day Master in Ba Zi terms. In general, the Day Master describes around 70 percent of a person's psychology. The Day Master explains the person's behavioral attributes in any given situation with other people, and also how the person is looking at the world and feels about the world and himself.

In addition to a personal element that is the foundation of the Day Master, we also have a polarity to the element that can be either yin or yang. This polarity is very interesting, because it explains two ways in which an element, and hence a persona, can express itself. Take for example a yang fire person versus a yin fire person. Since they both are of the fire element, they have a lot of common characteristics. For example, they can be warm and friendly, generous and passionate. But they also have the tendencies of becoming lonely and being very emotional. In contrast, the yang fire person is more extreme in their behavior and will take much more space than a yin fire person. In addition, a yin fire person will have a much more subtle way of telling people things, while the yang fire person will not be so refined.

Ba Zi (eight characters or eight palaces) consists of eight elements—from now on called characters—with their different polarities. And these eight characters are divided into two rows and four pillars:

Tian Gan (Heavenly Stems)				
Di Zhi (Earthly Branches)				

The upper row is called the Tian Gan (Heavenly Stems) and the lower row is called the Di Zhi (Earthly Branches). The Tian Gan represents what you as a person have been given by the heavens as attributes, and it is also here that the Day Master resides.

The Di Zhi, on the other hand, is what your incarnation on earth has at their disposal or, put another way, how your incarnation interacts with the world. In general, it is more interesting to understand your Di Zhi since it has much more to do with your daily life.

The four pillars are four columns that contain one character for the Tian Gan and one for the Di Zhi. The four pillars are known from left to the right as the Hour pillar, Day pillar, Month pillar and Year pillar, respectively. In the Tian Gan of the Day pillar you find your Day Master.

Tian Gan (Heavenly Stems)	HOUR	DAY	MONTH	YEAR
Di Zhi (Earthly Branches)				

This Ba Zi map shows a structure that details a person's psychological profile. In each of the palaces, we will have an element with its specific polarity. Each box will in itself have a certain amount of information with regard to its position in the four pillars, but also in relationship to which element and polarity it has. In addition, every palace interacts with other palaces in the same pillar or neighboring pillars. Also, each palace has more subtle interactions with palaces that are not adjacent to each other. Even though the Ba Zi map looks simple, it is far from being so—it is a combinatorial masterpiece of the human psyche.

Let us here give a short overview of the Ba Zi map. This will make it easier to follow when we start to go into the map in more detail and in its interpretation. The first thing we need to realize about the map is that it is of course specific to every person. And this is actually explained in the names of the pillars. In each pillar you will have elements with polarities specific to the person's hour, day, month and year of birth.

The next layer of interpreting the map is that it shows the dominant pillar with regard to one's age. This means that during the different stages of our mortal life we will have new Tian Gan and Di Zhi combinations that we can say will work as our Day Master for now. This is actually quite easy to see in the personalities of children and how they develop before adulthood. As they go through different stages, their personality is actually a little different. They have their core which does not change, but they are still influenced by things that make them different from what they were at an earlier age. This is where the pillar of that certain age comes into play. Another interesting function that a pillar has regarding a person's age is that it also changes the total picture of the map in terms of understanding age-related questions.

We can also look at the Ba Zi map from the core of our profile to the more superficial or least personal aspects of our person. This would be to read the map from the Hour pillar (innermost traits) to the Year pillar (outermost traits). For example, as a human being we have different layers of intimacy in terms of how we relate to colleagues, friends, family and spouse. We just behave differently towards people depending upon which social circle they belong to in our lives. People we do not know will be dominated by the characteristics of our Year pillar, while colleagues will be more prone to interact with our Month pillar, for example. And in contrast, there is always the deepest part of us that we do not share with anyone, and that would be represented by our Hour pillar.

Another aspect that we can understand from the Ba Zi map is actually how we perceive our self with regard to our own spiritual development, relationships and goals in life.

As you can see, there is so much that can be understood from the Ba Zi map. You just need to understand in detail what each pillar and box tell you by themselves and in all the possible combinations they can exist in.

As a general rule for interpreting the Ba Zi map, we can say the following: each situation that either is between you and another person, or you with yourself, can be divided into four levels (the pillars) depending upon the depth of the situation (with hour being the innermost level). The boxes in that level will then give you an explanation of how a situation can be resolved in terms of the person you are.

This is the structure of the Ba Zi map (four pillars and two rows). And it is from this map that we learn how to discern personal traits. You will also see that from this map you will immediately get a general understanding of people that will amaze you, but you will also find that the map is a very practical tool for resolving issues.

CHAPTER 2

Ba Zi

The Eight Characters

Ba Zi, or the eight characters (sometimes referred to as the eight palaces), provides us with an understanding of our deepest secrets that are shown in our outward behavior. The methodology rests on a multidimensional meaning that has many areas of application, from understanding ourselves in relationship to ourselves, to our relationship and interaction with other people. In addition, there are numerous other applications. Essentially, Ba Zi reveals our tendencies in life.

As with all Daoist tools and practices, using Ba Zi is of utmost importance, and treating it as just a piece of interesting information is not valuable. We need to actually *use* Ba Zi to understand a situation and act on it.

The table below gives the basic outline of Ba Zi:

	Hour	Day	Month	Year
Tian Gan (Heavenly Stems)		Day Master		
Di Zhi (Earthly Branches)				

The Day Master is the day palace of the heavenly stem. It is a very important palace and we will use it in many comparisons and interpretations.

The Day Master is who we believe we are, and understanding it reveals 70 percent of our personality. In later sections, we will look at the strength of the Day Master. This will give us valuable information in regard to being able to understand our personality, because time will affect a weak Day Master and the information it gives will not be enough.

There are three levels to Ba Zi:

1. *Who we are.* Our deep personality has tendencies which are given from birth and which we cannot change very much. Moreover, it is not always very practical to try to change them. Knowing our tendencies might enable us to prepare better for life events, but essentially it shows who we really are. However, when we have this understanding of ourselves, we can change how we see the world.

2. *How we see the world.* Because of who we are, we will see the world in a specific way.

3. *How we interact with the world.* When we know who we deeply are and how we interact in the world, we have the power to change how we do this.

These three levels are the Heaven, Man and Earth levels. It is important that we understand these, and the fact that they interact.

For the foundation of your own Ba Zi and that of others, you need to understand who you really are. The real basis for this are the ten Day Masters (the ten Tian Gan). These will be explained in more detail later, but in short they are the five elements, with yin and yang polarity.

Understanding the palaces

In this section, we will explore a few different ways to look at Ba Zi and how it affects our life. What we want to develop is a feel for the subject, and not just a regurgitation of information. As mentioned earlier, using it as a practical method will help us develop this more intuitive feeling that we are looking for.

The first thing to look at, and this is a traditional view, is how the columns relate to different stages of a person's life. The table below gives a more detailed description:

Hour	Retirement (52 and above)	The time when we stop being productive and we start reflecting on our life.
Day	Adulthood (35–51)	When we are responsible and independent in our own life. This is after a marriage, having a baby or separating financially from the family.
Month	Adolescence (18–34)	Friends, siblings and other people will shape how we will be as an adult—the time when we construct our individuality. It is a time when we want to know things. In addition, it is a time when we realize that not everybody is perfect, even family and ourselves.
Year	Childhood (17 and below)	The time when we have the "mommy and daddy" image and are completely dependent on our parents. Even if our childhood was bad, we remember it as good.

If a person follows a natural progression, then by the age of 40 they should be independent and mostly influenced by the Day pillar. However, someone might not get to adulthood because they are still dependent on their parents financially or in some other way and therefore will be influenced by the Month pillar more than normal. How the pillars relate and how they affect each other will be looked at in more detail later.

Here are a few more examples:

		Tian Gan	Di Zhi
Hour	Inside the home	Our children, us. The inside of us. The things we do not want to share. The Nei Hun.	Things that we do not know about ourselves, which are unclear.
Day		People we have a deep relationship with.	
Month	Outside the home	Parents and colleagues. We do not share intimate things with them.	
Year		Grandparents and outside life. The people we know but don't care what they say about us.	

More on ourselves:

	Tian Gan	Di Zhi
Hour *Spiritual*	The relationship with the higher (Shen). Messages we will receive. Spirits and angels. The quality and the capacity to listen to it. If we have yang earth or yang metal, our spiritual side is blocked. This will hinder us from reaching spirituality. However, this is different for practitioners. The practice gives us short cuts to see things differently. If there is no spiritual practice or a structured practice then we will feel pressure and be stuck. Felt as a fight and tension and not as an open canal! The capacity to listen to the spiritual side. Intuition. Connection with Yuan Shen. Can come by itself.	Deep grounding of our spirituality. Our ability to connect. Aspiration. The deep things we want in life. The relationship with the Gui. Deep meaning from practice. Conscious dream practice. Cannot come by itself.
Day *Relationships*	Represents us, and us towards others. Towards people in our home. The interaction between the Day Master and earthly branch gives us our tendencies for relationships. The good and the bad. What we look for in a relationship. The problems of what we look for. What we will expect from the other.	Relationship to other people or wife/husband. How we behave in our home behind closed doors.

Month Emotional	What we do with emotions. Our emotional filter. The way we have relationships with others. The way we judge things in our mental mind! How others see the relationship with us. How we adapt with our friends. The way we filter things with our perception of the world. What we do with the emotions. The way we show our emotions to people; how we share them.	How we digest emotions. Some problems will always be there and not digested. Deep relationship with parents. All problems with parents. Fuel of our Day Master. The month of our birth. Season aspects. What drives us emotionally.
Year Material	What we will do and produce in the world. Our hobbies. What we show to people. The job we choose and what we aspire to.	Family heritage. The ancestral link. Our health capital. What we got, our *jing*. See how it relates to our Day Master. Imbalance in health will be felt. What we feel outside with people.

The earthly branch (Di Zhi) should feed the heavenly stem; however, sometimes the heavenly stem will stop the realization of the earthly branch, or vice versa. This is a very interesting relationship and we will look at it in more detail later.

What we also need to have in the back of our minds is that the earthly branch is a realization of heaven, so inside the earthly branch we have a heavenly stem.

Ba Zi regarding work:

	Tian Gan	Di Zhi
Hour	Helps us do things. The things that help us to work.	People who we control that we help. They also give us our drive. They push us to do more but we don't tell them.
Day	ME!	Assistant or direct associates. If we are the boss it will be our right-hand man.
Month	Close colleagues who carry us, and friends at work who help us.	People who give us good ideas. They give us the path. Mentors. The good boss.
Year	Colleagues, boss or people we interact with and work with.	Drive. The fuel for work.

Ba Zi and Feng Shui

With Ba Zi we have facing and sitting. We need this when we want to combine Ba Zi with Feng Shui:

- Hour: sitting point → Di Zhi
- Year: facing point → Tian Gan
- In the middle, you have a combination of Nei Hun and Wai Hun.

Yin and yang

One of the first things we look for in Ba Zi is balance. That is, the balance of yin and yang, but also that of the elements. What we do not want is to think that, for example, we need more yang in our Ba Zi so that we start doing more yang things when our Ba Zi has already more than enough yang. Each of the characters (palaces) will have a polarity, yin or yang. We will measure the balance of yin and yang and see what we need to do.

Yin/yang is so huge that, if we were very good at dealing with it, we would not need anything else. However, it is so complex that we need the laws of the five elements.

The five elements

For Ba Zi it is very important to know the theory of the five elements. The five cycles to remember are:

1. *Creation.* Water → wood → fire → earth → metal → water.

2. *Controlling.* It is healthy: metal → wood → earth → water → fire → metal.

3. *Insulting.* The reverse of controlling: metal ← wood ← earth ← water ← fire ← metal.

4. *Exhausting.* The reverse of creation: water ← wood ← fire ← earth ← metal ← water.

5. *Reinforcing.* The same element reinforces the same element. For example, if you have two fires it is reinforced in Ba Zi, but if you have six fires it is too much.

Out of these, cycles 1, 2 and 4 are the most important to remember.

Note: We are looking for balance in Ba Zi, so we want a balance of the elements.

CHAPTER 3

The Heavenly Stems

The five elements and their polarity form the basis of Ba Zi. It is thus important that we have a good understanding of them regarding the eight palaces. Therefore, in this chapter, we will look at the ten heavenly stems, ranging from the general to the more polarity-specific tendencies, and consider the positives and negatives as they relate to work and training.

Wood

The wood element is about growth and continuous development. There is also strength in the growth. Wood is an energy that wants to go everywhere.

General

Wood people are progressive, persevering and stable. They are straight and clear in their manner, which is good because this means they will be honest. However, it is very difficult to change what they believe. This also relates to persuasion, though they might change over time. Wood people are sentimental and do not want to be away from their roots, particularly where they were born or grew up. Even if they clash with their family or fall out of love with their country they will always come back; or they will move very far away but re-create their home or neighborhood in the new place. Stability and not moving are particular tendencies of wood people. As a result of their roots they are steady and we can lean on them for help. They will always be somewhat successful; indeed, it is very difficult for wood people not to be successful.

Positives

Wood people are good at communicating and transmitting. Therefore, they also want to be the person who can explain things and be a messenger to other people. They are kind, tender, ambitious, audacious, optimistic, enthusiastic and even romantic. The ability to see things from a broader perspective or to see the big picture are other positive qualities of such people. Because of this, they are open to many things. Some qualities are based on their ability to "know who they are," such as being able to judge or taking the initiative. Guided by their gut feeling, they will not act if it is not right. We mentioned earlier that it is difficult to make them change their mind; however, this is possible if the change goes in the direction they want to go in. We can count on wood people as they are honest and ethical and have a good memory. A challenge is always welcome, though if they do not like advice, then they have to think about it. Having a survival instinct is a known trait; and they are good at developing projects, solving problems and planning because they know where to go. Wood people have ideas, imagination, creativity and the desire to create. They have a good capacity to learn, going deep into an occupation. In addition, as soon as they want to discover who they are, they can examine their spirituality. In addition, they have an artistic mind, and mobility of the body and mind. They are quick, and therefore they need movement.

Negatives

Wood people can be frustrated, irritated and impatient. They need to be recognized and can have a low self-image. Because of the growing energy of wood, everything in life seems to be small; or they are impatient because they are not already where they want to be. Since they expand everywhere, they do not want their development to be blocked or to go too slowly; if that is the case, then they become nervous and irritated, or even depressed. This means they are always in a hurry, always in an "I want, I want" mood, possibly leading towards anger and rage. In addition, wood people are not easily satisfied and try to forget about events, because they do not want to see reality. They can be aggressive, menacing and unfriendly, have a tendency to want to be right, cannot delegate, and are sometimes moody and confused. Moreover, they have a tendency to be stuck in their beliefs and can stop other people from developing so that they can develop better themselves. On one side they can have low self-esteem; on the other they can feel that they are so much more important than other people. They will "kill" everybody in order to go towards what they want to do, and would rather destroy than rebuild.

A situation might easily hurt or vex them. They are susceptible and stubborn, look for confrontation or to be provoking, like to upset people, and are very demanding. It is difficult for them to predict what they want, and they do not like advice or orders. Wood people have the tendency to be too emotional, straight or psychologically rigid. They will not say "thank you" and will be jealous. Their insecurity might also be because they do not know where they want to go. At least most of the time, people have to adapt to them rather than them adapting to other people.

Training

Wood people need strong muscles and tendons. In addition, they need to keep their neck, shoulder and trapezius muscles very flexible. Tai Ji and any kind of conscious walking will be good for this. Other recommended training should be yin in nature, such as the Dao. They also need to take care not to eat too much acidic food.

Work

Architecture, Woodworking, Development and communication, Education and teaching, Research, Psychology, Human research, Rational therapy, Philosophy, Medicine (mostly exotic medicine), Re-education, Optics and eyes, Herbs and biology, Work involving the earth, Plants and flowers, Botany, Forest ranger, Fashion, Hairdresser, Clothes design, Writing, Bookselling, Media, Documentation, Biotech, Music, Singing, Poetry, Ecology, Energy linked to the wind or wood, Renewable technology, Political strategy.

Jia (yang wood) qualities

Jia people will be flexible but also stubborn and rigid. They will stand their ground and stick to their beliefs. Whereas yin wood needs yang wood, yang wood does not need yin wood. Yang wood people are good, but they can easily upset others because of their straight and righteous manner. In addition, they may not be very tactful or are just too outspoken. They can be boring and conservative, but they are the best people to rely on and have a relationship with because they are steady and clear. Because they are very smart, they have a great capacity for learning. Like a rigid tree, they will always continue to grow and progress. They will never stop. On the other hand, they do not like ambition. They are very thorough, and they will always be successful once they find out what they want to do. We can never stop the successful growth of a yang wood person. They are straightforward people, but a little obsessive. As they are loyal, you can charge into war with them. The yang wood person might not look sentimental but they are very much so—sometimes too much.

- Famous people: Napoleon, Bruce Lee, Richard Branson (Virgin Records, etc.), Ralph Lauren.

Yi (yin wood) qualities

Yi people are survivalists, and are flexible and subtle. They are attached to others and need yang wood. They are pretty, soft, gentle and elegant and like the finer things of life. Yi men will be talented and Yi women beautiful, elegant and refined. Yin wood people will be smart, witty and adaptive. Life is about survival, and they will even do bad things to survive. They do not have the straightness of Jia (yang wood). However, they are very difficult to break (like bamboo). As with wood, in general they like to expand, so because of this they like to be everywhere, but they do not like to be controlled by other people. They are patient and straightforward in their behavior, but primarily they want to survive. In addition, being pushed around is something that they do not tolerate. Yin wood people need some fire for talent and happiness because they will sometimes be locked into their own minds.

- Famous people: Bill Clinton.

Fire
Life, being alive, and the basic energy of survival—this is fire.

General
Fire people are warm, friendly, expressive, passionate, loving, compassionate and empathetic.

Positives
Some positive aspects of fire people are politeness, good manners, patience, generosity, willingness to help others, passion and intelligence. They are illuminating and give light to other people's lives, stimulating people. In addition, they like to extend their knowledge to other people. Like the sun, they have good powers of attraction. Often they will also have a good appearance and like to be attractive. Since fire is about living, they will aim to be

happy and do what they can to achieve this. As a result, they know how to live and do not say no to partying. Fire people need to do something important and contribute. Moreover, they need to show on the outside what is on the inside. They are expansive, dynamic, action oriented, productive and spontaneous and will express themselves strongly. In addition, they will talk loudly, do things, explain, and might even make a discovery. Fire people are attentive to other people, bringing people together, and they can mediate. They have mental clarity, are lucid, good teachers and can easily absorb knowledge. Therefore, they learn quickly and are very intelligent. People of the fire element like things to stay the same and, similar to the sun, will never lack power and can have an intense nature. The more you go against them, the more they will come back. Fire is about dynamic movement and power, but also about warmth and attention. Fire people like attention.

Negatives

The negative aspects of fire people are that they are lonely and do not like surprises. They will be independent as long as people are dependent on them. As fire is the only element that can consume itself and therefore needs resources, fire people need to feed on something, otherwise they will feed on themselves. Fire people can be egocentric, attached to things, jealous and destructive (self-destructive), and have difficulties seeing things through to the end. Moreover, they can also do too many things at the same time. Being the sun, they are more fragile than you think, and feelings and emotions can consume them. In the end, they can also be very superficial because they can attract more people that way.

Training
Fire people need to have a good balance between mind and spirit. In addition, they need to breathe; the breath will feed the fire and quieten it. And they need to learn to do nothing.

Work
Metaphysics, Religion and spirituality (especially for yin fire), Technology, Aeronautics, Chemistry, Petroleum industry, Electricity and electronics, Informatics and telecommunications industry, Weapons (Bing: yang fire), Fire service, Esthetics, Public relations, publicity and media, Performance arts and dance, Art, Lighting and sound, Communication, Foods industry, Barkeeper (but would drink all the alcohol!).

Bing (yang fire) qualities
Bing people are regarded as the only one or like the sun. They are solitary; they like routine and for things to stay the same. They do not like surprises and are not very adaptable. As the sun, they are very independent and will never be destroyed, but will be there if people need them. However, they have to be at the center of things, the most important person that people look at—though do not get too close or they will burn you. Even if they live a simple and sheltered life, they will influence or touch people around them. Yang fire people are talented, hardworking

and confident. They like to teach and show people things, but might not be subtle in the way they teach because they think they know best. Like a volcano, yang fire has lots of emotion that will burst out all the time. Yang fire people will get angry and scream, even resorting to violence if needed. Finally, they will be exceptional actors and performers.

- Famous people: Steve Jobs, Nelson Mandela.

Ding (yin fire) qualities

Yin fire is candle light or a torch. As fire people, they need something to feed their fire (resources). A candle is fragile and can be sentimental, but it lights up, so therefore they learn and teach fast and are like a sponge regarding knowledge, but will in turn burn out quickly. They are open to others because they always guide people. Thus, they will know people and consequently will always be suspicious since they know how people work and function. Yin fire people are generous and benevolent (kind) and will always help others. However, they can do too much and, because of this, they will be good martyrs. Leaders by nature, they will easily become so even without people realizing it. People will just start following them. They are excellent motivators, but the fire is fragile and they can easily destroy themselves by giving too much. Yin fire people get bored if they do not have one clear thing to do. And on a few occasions and for a small amount of time the Ding can create a huge fire bigger than the Bing.

- Famous people: Tony Robbins (motivational speaker), Walt Disney, Phil Knight (co-founder of Nike).

Earth

General

Earth people do not have it easy because the main thing for them is silence, and this is inside. Silence is golden, they would say. Slow, quiet and thorough would be a way to describe earth people. With their silence, they are good at keeping secrets. However, things will take time, and getting information is like digging for gold. When they finally say something, they will go into very little detail. One thing about earth is that yin and yang are very different.

Positives

The positive aspects of earth people are balance, stability, confidence, sincerity, respectability, viability and receptivity. They are often old-fashioned, preferring home and staying there, are sentimental, strong but slow, and will resist through the passage of time. If things please the earth person, they will not move anymore and therefore they need to be stimulated to move. In line with their preference to be at home, earth people also like protection (security), shelter and that things stay as they are for a long time. They are sentimental ("it was better before" kind of thinking), have a very good sense of family and home, can be very devoted and are very welcoming. Earth people will nourish those around them; they are the first to help and are good at organizing their life. They know instinctively how to go to the heart of a matter and, because of that, they are very grounded. This also leads to a good sense of balance and harmony. Earth people will help others with their fertility; they like to touch (massage). They are also empathetic, good mediators and coaches and just good at doing things. With their mental capacity, they will think a lot, concentrate a lot and memorize things. They assimilate quite easily and will look into things to understand them better. Earth people love to do familiar activities and are very sharing.

Negatives

A negative aspect of earth people is that they accumulate not just things but also emotions. They will be confused, inattentive, distracted, worried and anxious, and are obsessive thinkers.

Earth people will also be immobile if they are comfortable or they do too much. They can easily end up just sitting on the couch doing nothing and waiting for things to happen, even if nothing happens. In other words, they are lazy and slow. They will also have the same immobility of mind, resulting in very fixed ideas and lack of creativity. Other negative aspects are that they can be manipulated into doing bad things. They will be mean, negligent and nostalgic, turn to self-pity and isolate themselves. Being comfortable results in the love of habits, and because of this they will be discouraged easily.

Training

Earth people need to walk a lot (move) and to be in retreat or to be alone. Resting is also important, as is working on the breath! They also need to push themselves regarding physical activity.

Work

Real estate, Insurance, Security, Natural resources, Construction (e.g. masons or builders), Ceramics, Sculptures, Antiquities and selling art, Gardening, Archeology, Geology, Farming, Food industry, Teaching physical education, Occidental medicine, Massage, Helping and curing people, Human resources, Social work, Helping and working with animals, Stone work, Mining, Archiving, Tourism industry.

Wu (yang earth) qualities

Yang earth is about the home, the familiar, protection and shelter. It is also about things that make you slow. An image for yang earth is the mountain. Yang earth people are solid, trustworthy, stubborn, inflexible, unyielding and very confident, will make good soldiers and guardians, and will be one's best friends because they will be there for us. Yang earth people value their honor, reputation and what they say. Whatever they do, it will take time. They are tough on the outside and full of emotions on the inside. They tend to be best friends and good parents because they have a real concern for other people. These will be the people who defend society.

Ji (yin earth) qualities

Yin earth is the master of ego! Yin earth people really think they are smart and that they know best. However, they are very resourceful and multi-talented. This is the only Day Master that can do everything in life. Yin earth is the image of the fertile soil; yin earth people will be neutering, nourishing and very productive and they can pretty much produce what they want. They will be good at listening and saying yes while doing and saying things behind our back. In addition, they are very good at taking a situation and moving it towards what they want. Moreover, they love to discuss and have arguments and just talking for talking's sake, which makes them good at politics. Yin earth is the mental mind, and therefore they will always analyze and think about everything that can happen and why people do things, even if nothing has happened. This is good for research and study but unnecessary for many other things. They make very good religious people. We just send them on their path and they will do it; however, they need to focus on a higher goal in life or they will never gain money. In addition, if they are put in a situation where they are not certain, they will ask many questions. As with all earth characteristics, things take time. They are also very sensitive to water because it carries disease and provides dispersion; despite this, they have very good health.

- Famous people: Barack Obama, Abraham Lincoln.

Metal

General

Metal people are tough and resilient but altruistic and humane. In addition, they need things to be fair, just and right.

Positives

A positive aspect of metal is that it is basic ego—the capacity to choose and judge, and the ability to cut through. Metal people are also to the fore in decision making, altruism (selflessness), justice (law), pride and organization (planning), but will also be animalistic, instinctive, combative, courageous and clear. Metal people will never forget anything; if we have done something wrong, they will make us pay. They will also be straight, practical, proud, strong (resilient), loyal, elegant, smart, clever, structured, precise and careful.

Other qualities are that metal people can make others change, and they always try to do better, seeking perfection. Furthermore, they look for quality and like to express themselves creatively. This sense of creativity comes not only from metal but also the interaction with fire, so they need to have fire in their Ba Zi for this. They will be law abiding, very constant, make good defensive strategists, conformist (traditional), very romantic and strong on distribution and control. Driving is about decision making, and consequently they will be good drivers. A metal person will be a master of what he is doing, good at cleaning up things, organizing files and bringing things together. Lastly, they love pleasure, but in a smart way.

Negatives

Metal people can be brutish, barbarian, intolerant, perfectionistic and authoritarian. They need to be tamed and forged because they give 100 percent all of the time. Furthermore, they will think a lot (old memories) and can withdraw into themselves and want to be alone. Metal is related to the lungs, which is related to sadness; therefore they can be very sad and cry over nothing! They might look strong but can be very fragile. Other negative aspects are that they might not like change, they will say no all the time, and be psychologically rigid. Other characteristics might be difficulty in forgiving people, while having a bad memory while thinking that it is good. They can destroy everything just because of some little thing. In addition, they might also not take care of things and be obsessed with a future that is never real.

Training

For training and practice, metal people should do mind work (Shen Gong) and always walk around, not staying inside. They should never smoke, due to the relation of metal to the lungs in Chinese medicine.

Work

Justice, Law, Police and army, Metal work including jewelry, Mechanics, Anything precise, Medicine (surgery), Interior design or similar where they make things look better, Finances, Banking, Accountancy, Money, Martial arts, Anything metal-related, Maintenance, Inspection, Electronics.

Geng (yang metal) qualities

Yang metal is like a heavy ax. Pure strength and brutal, yang metal is the toughest of all the Day Masters. Furthermore, yang metal people easily withstand hardship and go on directly and powerfully without thinking. Consequently, some power is needed to forge and refine them. In life, they will be happier if they can deal with big problems. Therefore, problems such as confronting life and death are easy, but small things are not. This might get them depressed. Metal is about decision making and action and that is especially true for yang metal people; so if we help them too much, they will not like it. They are also very hands-on, use tools and get their hands dirty. This roughness of yang metal people means also that they are often impolite, brash and impulsive. On the other hand, they will be playful with a little bit of craziness. These people are the old stubborn warriors who will not take advice. Making decisions is one of their key characteristics, which works very well for chaotic and difficult situations but not as well for simple trivial tasks. As a result they need to believe in big principles or they will not function properly. Even with this hardness, they need people around them, especially family and people they like. In addition, they will not forget us!

- Famous people: Queen Elizabeth, Muhammad Ali, Margaret Thatcher.

Xin (yin metal) qualities

Yin metal, unlike yang metal, is worked metal, a piece of jewelry. It is about appearance, beauty, artistic expression and attention. Yin metal people love attention and like to grab it. But in their ability to shine they need success, and this is only possible if they have fire (genius) or water (wisdom) in their Ba Zi. This will give them abilities. Without these abilities, they can be depressed. Sometimes they want the ability, power or authority so badly that they lose themselves in it so that they do not have it. When they have abilities, they are very talented; they like doing things, but sometimes get caught up and do not finish them. But when they see a solution they grab it and use it at once. Yin metal people are very sentimental and value family and relationships. Compared to yang metal people, they are much more easily influenced by others. They are proud (the most proud Day Master), jealous, noisy and difficult to handle. In addition, they are tough but nicer in character than yang metal people. And they will forget us!

- Famous people: Gordon Ramsay (chef), Sacha Baron Cohen (actor).

Water
General

Water is about wisdom and intelligence. It is the capacity to use knowledge. Water people are adaptive and imaginative and the keepers of secrets. However, they need be in motion to be happy.

Positives

A positive aspect of water is that it is the source of power and wisdom of human beings. Water is knowledge, devotion, determination (will-power), sentimentality, introspection and resilience. Water people have the ability to go in every direction, but they need to be focused. With this innate knowledge, and ability to recognize love in others, they will easily nourish and teach people. They will have good communication skills, not just towards others but inward as well. Their minds will be active, and they will have good memory and concentration and be curious. Furthermore, they will think before they act and look at things for a long time. However, they will always be in motion. They are mysterious (like a mystery), focused, deep, complex, very careful and intuitive. Generally, they will have plenty of possibilities, be fragile but strong, and always find a solution. With their ability to teach, they will also be good with children and students and will help people. Water people also have bad habits (for example, being liars).

Negatives

The negative aspects of water people are that they are not very centered and are dispersed, unstable and restless. They will often be fearful, distressed, phobic, nervous and stressed. Furthermore, they can be depressed, emotional, vulnerable and stagnant (doing nothing). They can also be silent and introverted and think too much. They can be slow (but not as slow as earth people), complain and easily lose energy. Often they will do things the wrong way.

They will not express their emotions or show what is on the inside. In addition, they can be impractical and difficult to approach.

Training

Water people need to move and do yang-type exercises, for example Gong Fu. Too much static work will not be good for them.

Work

All work related to the sea, such as being in the Navy or being a sailor, Selling and buying (retail), Postal work, Moving things, Removals, Tourism, Analysis, Strategy, Journalism, Transportation, Anything to help creativity, Hygiene and cleaning, Politics (because they are good at lying and selling), Spirituality and meditation, Astronomy, Hydrology.

Ren (yang water) qualities

Yang water is a tsunami, never stopping. It is a huge power that drives in one direction. Yang water people are very intelligent, but they might not seem that way sometimes because they go so fast in one direction and do not stop to think. Furthermore, they can be unstoppable as soon as they choose where to go. They have the capacity to drive people. Water people are extrovert, outspoken, quick-tempered, forceful and brash. In their forceful motion they might get lost and therefore become unfocused and get distracted. They move in all directions but can also change their direction very easily. They are very opportunistic, adventurous and courageous. In their confusion, they can lose track of what they believe in and behave in a mischievous and manipulating way. However, they are deeply honest and straight. Finally, yang water people will be successful.

- Famous people: Bill Gates, Queen Victoria, Charles Merrill (Merrill Lynch Wealth Management).

Gui (yin water) qualities

Yin water is mist. Yin water people look passive but are not. A mist engulfs us without us realizing it and suddenly we have signed the contract. Although they do not look like teachers, they will talk and then we will realize that we have learned something. Yin water is also about intuition and instinct. Yin water people have lots on their mind and can be very dreamy and fantasize about things. On the other hand, they are imaginative and have the capacity to see the big picture. Sometimes they are paranoid and can be perverted and sadistic. They are nourishing, calm, slow-moving and interacting. They can look timid and emotional but still be strong. Yin water people solve things in a soft way and will be very romantic. Their softness makes them good with children.

- Famous people: Stephen King, Jamie Oliver (chef).

CHAPTER 4

The Earthly Branches

The twelve animals

Now that we have talked a little bit about the heavenly stems, in this chapter we look at the manifestation they have on earth, the earthly branches. The earthly branches, referred to as the twelve animals, make up the lower row in the eight palaces. We are not actually concerned with the animal image because the names are not the correct Chinese names for the animals. They are more important than the heavenly stems and, furthermore, they have rhythm and season. The animals are as follows:

Spring	Yang wood	Yin	Tiger	Feb 4–Mar 5
	Yin wood	Mao	Rabbit	Mar 6–Apr 4
	Yang earth	Chen	Dragon	Apr 5–May 5
Summer	Yin fire	Si	Snake	May 6–Jun 5
	Yang fire	Wu	Horse	Jun 6–Jul 6
	Yin earth	Wei	Goat	Jul 7–Aug 7
Fall	Yang metal	Shen	Monkey	Aug 8–Sep 7
	Yin metal	You	Rooster	Sep 8–Oct 7
	Yang earth	Xu	Dog	Oct 8–Nov 6

Winter	Yin water	Hai	Pig	Nov 7–Dec 6
	Yang water	Zi	Rat	Dec 7–Jan 5
	Yin earth	Chou	Ox	Jan 6–Feb 3

We need to know the animals and their Chinese names. One simple way to memorize the Chinese names is by the seasons:

- Spring: Yin, Mao, Chen
- Summer: Si, Wu, Wei
- Fall: Shen, You, Xu
- Winter: Hai, Zi, Chou.

Note: We also need to learn the heavenly stems as well. Therefore, in total we will have 22 Chinese names to learn.

An example

This basic structure of Ba Zi provides us with some information regarding a person. Below we give an example of Ba Zi for a person born on 23 November 2013 at 10 o'clock.

	Hour	Day	Month	Year
Tian Gan	DING Yin fire	GUI Yin water	GUI Yin water	GUI Yin water
Di Zhi	SI Snake Yin fire	SI Snake Yin fire	HAI Pig Yin water	SI Snake Yin fire

The first thing we can see is that there is a serious imbalance of yin and yang in this Ba Zi. It only consists of yin elements. Furthermore, these elements are just fire and water. What does this mean? It means the person's thinking will be in conflict. This is bad! So, already we know something about this person—life will be hard for them.

Hidden stems

There is more information connected to the earthly branches. Each of the earthly branches can have one to three hidden heavenly stems depending on the earthly branch. These hidden stems consist of one major stem and zero to two supporting stems. In each of the hidden stems you have the root of your Day Master. This is very important! These hidden stems are the human part of us, which comes from our family, country of birth and so on. Moreover, they will help balance the Ba Zi.

The energy of the hidden stems is dependent on where the earthly branch is in the season. Consequently, branches at the beginning will be in growth. The cardinals are in the middle of the season, and the graveyards are at the end:

- *The growth.* The growth is at the beginning of the season. The energy is growing. The branch will have 2–3 hidden stems because they have more energy and give more information.

- *The cardinals.* The cardinals are in the middle of the season. The energy is there but it is not weak. Most of the branches have one hidden stem, except Wu (Horse), which has two.

- *The graveyards.* The graveyards are at the end of the season. The energy is going down.

	Earthly branches			Hidden heavenly stems		
The growth	Yin	Tiger	Yang wood	Jia – Yang wood	Bing – Yang fire	Wu – Yang earth
	Shen	Monkey	Yang metal	Geng – Yang metal	Ren – Yang water	Wu – Yang earth
	Si	Snake	Yin fire	Bing – Yang fire	Wu – Yang earth	Geng – Yang metal
	Hai	Pig	Yin water	Ren – Yang water	Jia – Yang wood	
The cardinals	Zi	Rat	Yang water	Gui – Yin water		
	Wu	Horse	Yang fire	Ding – Yin fire	Ji – Yin earth	
	Mao	Rabbit	Yin wood	Yi – Yin wood		
	You	Rooster	Yin metal	Xin – Yin metal		
The graveyards	Chen	Dragon	Yang earth	Wu – Yang earth	Yi – Yin wood	Gui – Yin water
	Xu	Dog	Yang earth	Wu – Yang earth	Xin – Yin metal	Ding – Yin fire
	Chou	Ox	Yin earth	Ji – Yin earth	Gui – Yin water	Xin – Yin metal
	Wei	Goat	Yin earth	Ji – Yin earth	Ding – Yin fire	Yi – Yin wood

An example

	Day column
Tian Gan	Gui (Yin water)
Di Zhi	Si (Yin fire)
Hidden stem	Bing (Yang fire)

Since there is yin water in the stems and yang fire as the hidden stem, this is not so good.

Determining the strength of the Day Master

It is important to determine the strength of the Day Master because if it is strong then we will have all its qualities, but if it is weak we will have all the negative aspects of it. There are three parts to determining the strength of the Day Master:

1. Season (70%)

2. Root (25%)

3. Formation (5%).

The percentages give the importance of the three parts. Therefore, timing (season) is the most important, while formation is the least important.

Season

Each of the heavenly stems has one element and one polarity. Each of them will then have a perfect fit in the season (see the table below). Here are some examples:

- Example I
  - Day Master: Ding (yin fire)
  - Born: Summer, Si (Snake) yin fire
  - Comment: Si is in the growth of the hidden stems and is therefore very good.
- Example II
  - Day Master: Bing (yang fire)
  - Born: Summer, Wu (Horse) yang fire
  - Comment: Here you do not want the energy to be growing because you are already the sun. Therefore, Wu is the best fit because it is in the cardinals of the hidden stems.

So, if you are wood you want to be born in the spring, likewise fire in the summer, metal in the fall and water in the winter. But for earth it doesn't matter too much because it will never be weak; it will always be medium strength.

Strength / Season	Dead	Very weak	Weak	Strong	Prosperous
Spring	Earth	Metal	Water	Fire	Wood
Summer	Metal	Water	Wood	Earth	Fire
Fall	Wood	Fire	Earth	Water	Metal
Winter	Fire	Earth	Metal	Wood	Water

Root

There are two kinds of root connected to the Day Master.

THE NORMAL

This is where the hidden stem of the day should be the same as the Day Master:

- Example I
  - Day Tian Gan: Ding (yin fire)
  - Day Di Zhi: Hai (yin water)
  - Hidden: yang water and yang wood
  - Comment: This might not look good because you think that yin fire is only supported by water. However, in the hidden stem there is also yang wood. Wood creates fire (cycle of creation). It is quite good but not great.
- Example II
  - Day Tian Gan: Ding (yin fire)
  - Day Di Zhi: Si (yin fire)
  - Hidden: yang fire
  - Comment: Here we see that yin fire is supported by yang fire, which is even better.

THE SECRET

This is where the hidden stem of the hour should be the same as the Day Master:

- Example:
  - Day Tian Gan: Ding (yin fire)
  - Hour Tian Gan: Bing (yang fire)
  - Hour Di Zhi: Wu (Horse, yang fire)
  - Hidden: yin fire and yin earth
  - Comment: This is really good.

Formation

Look at everything that supports the Day Master in the eight palaces and hidden stems.

Luck pillars

Luck pillars are about the period of time from your date of birth and a specific time in the future, even after death. If you miss elements or qualities in your Ba Zi with regard to doing something, you can look at the Luck pillars to find the right time to do them.

Finding the pillars

Take the month column of the Ba Zi. This will be the basis of the calculation of the Luck pillars.

We will start with ten pillars going from right to left. The month column we put to the right of the first Luck pillar. The Tian Gan and Di Zhi of the month gives us the starting point of setting the Tian Gan and Di Zhi of the Luck pillars.

The year column of the Ba Zi is either yin or yang. This will give us the order in which the Tian Gan and the Di Zhi are added for each column in the Luck pillars with regard to the gender of the person:

- Tian Gan: Jia, Yi, Bing, Ding, Wu, Ji, Geng, Xin, Ren and Gui

- Di Zhi: Yin, Mao, Chen, Si, Wu, Wei, Shen, You, Xu, Hai, Zi and Chou

- If man:
  - Yang: Right order. Jia → Gui
  - Yin: Reverse order. Gui → Jia
- If woman:
  - Yin: Right order. Jia → Gui
  - Yang: Reverse order. Gui → Jia
- *Note:* The starting point will be the Tian Gan or Di Zhi after the month column. For example, if the Tian Gan is Ding, then you start with Wu in the first column if it is in the right order, or Bing if it is in the reverse order. For the Di Zhi it will be that if we are Shen then we start with You in the right order, or Wei if it is in the reverse order.

Finding the age of the pillars:

- For this you need the ten-thousand-year calendar.
- Take the date of birth. The next day will be where we start counting, that is 1.
- We then count the days until the next change of the solar month.
- Divide this number by 3 and leave out the remainder. This will be the first number in the first pillar (a_1 in the table below).
- Then for each column, you add 10 years. This will be on top of the pillars.
- At the bottom there will also be a five-year interval. This is based on taking the age on top and adding 5.

		Tian Gan	Di Zhi	
	$a_{10}=a_9+10$			$a_{10}+5$
	$a_9=a_8+10$			a_9+5
	$a_8=a_7+10$			a_8+5
	$a_7=a_6+10$			a_7+5
	$a_6=a_5+10$			a_6+5
	$a_5=a_4+10$			a_5+5
	$a_4=a_3+10$			a_4+5
	$a_3=a_2+10$			a_3+5
	$a_2=a_1+10$			a_2+5
	a_1			a_1+5
Ba Zi	Month			
	Year			

Understanding the pillars

From the building of the pillars, we have ten-year intervals and five-year intervals. From the time of birth until a_1 age, the first Luck pillar will influence us. The Ba Zi will then not be four pillars but five: the four from the Ba Zi plus the first Luck pillar. We add this to the interpretation of Ba Zi.

Then from age a_1 until a_1+5 we will mostly be influenced by the element of the Tian Gan of the first pillar. Then from a_1+5 until a_2 the Di Zhi of the first pillar will influence us. Then from a_2 until a_2+5 the Tian Gan of the second pillar will influence us, and so on.

This means that your Ba Zi will always be five pillars and that no Ba Zi will always be bad. Therefore, timing is a big thing.

Note: If one of the Luck pillars is exactly the same as your birth pillars (hour, day, month or year), it means this is a time of change. The significance of this change depends on which column of the Ba Zi it is.

CHAPTER 5

Tools for Interpreting the Ba Zi

The five factors and the ten gods

The five factors are linked to the understanding of the cycle of creation and the cycle of control, while the ten gods add polarity (yin and yang).

The five factors

For the five factors we need to look at the cycle of creation and the cycle of control. We look at five factors in our lives and see the element linked to each. The five factors are:

1. Parallel/friends/brothers:
   - The parallel is us and the people that will be close to us—the people that we are close to.
   - *Element:* Same as the Day Master.

2. Work/output/children:
   - This what we produce—what we do for work. This will also be our capacity for doing things in the world.

- ° *Element:* This will be the element that our Day Master creates (produces).

3. Wealth/wife:

- ° Wealth is what we control—money and things that we own. This is not only money that we have produced but also money from our parents. However, this is not about whether or not we have money, but our relationship to it.
- ° *Element:* The element that our Day Master controls.

4. Influence/power/ghost officer:

- ° This is our power—the thing that controls us. It will also be our ability to touch people. What does control us is the greed for power and our wish to be important. In this factor parts of our shadows are present.
- ° *Element:* The element that controls our Day Master.

5. Resources/education/parents:

- ° Resources are the things that produce us—what makes or creates us. It is also our thinking and feeling. This will be from our own studies and research. This will give us our sense of happiness. That is why seeking knowledge and studying is so important because it produces us!
- ° *Element:* The element that creates (produces) the Day Master element.

The ten gods

The ten gods are the most important aspect of Ba Zi with regard to looking for specific information. As stated earlier, they are the five factors with polarity, hence the ten gods. The ten gods represent the relationship the heavenly stems have with the Day Master. Since this is about the heavenly stems, we will have three ten gods in the main eight mansions, but also we have to remember the hidden stems. Here we can have a number of ten gods depending on which of the stems we have. Remember that the hidden stems could range from one to three, depending on the earthly branch! There is a wealth of information with regard to them and we will consider only a condensed version of it here. The names are not important in themselves, but we need to know them so that we know which aspect they are.

Finding the ten gods

To find the ten gods we first need to look at our Day Master and see what element it is and what polarity it has. There are five groups of the gods, and therefore there will be two in each. These five groups are the five factors we presented earlier. In addition, the polarity of a god will be either the same or the opposite. For example, if our Day Master is yang wood (Jia) and we are comparing it with yin earth (Ji), then we know that wood controls earth (cycle of control)—therefore the ten god is in wealth. Moreover, as we readily see, they are of opposite polarity. Therefore, the ten god is Direct Wealth. Given below are the names of all of the ten gods:

1. Friends:
   ◦ Same polarity: Friends
   ◦ Opposite polarity: Rob Wealth
2. Work:
   ◦ Same polarity: Eating God
   ◦ Opposite polarity: Hurting Officer
3. Wealth:
   ◦ Same polarity: Indirect Wealth
   ◦ Opposite polarity: Direct Wealth
4. Influence:
   ◦ Same polarity: Seven Killings
   ◦ Opposite polarity: Direct Officer
5. Resources:
   ◦ Same polarity: Indirect Resource
   ◦ Opposite polarity: Direct Resource

For each of the ten gods there will be three different descriptions: a basic one, which we always read; and then there will be either a positive or a negative one. Whether a god is positive or negative depends on clashes and the stars—this will be discussed later.

Friends (Social Circles and Emotion)

- *Basic description.* The basic aspects of Friends individuals are that they will take initiative and be brave. They have trust in themselves and will look for people with the same values.

- *Positive description.* They are independent, honorable and strong-willed and will deal well with emotions. They will also have a good relationship with people.

- *Negative description.* The negative aspects of Friends individuals are being impulsive, having a big ego and people not understanding them. They will have problems with personal relationships and will be easily betrayed.

Rob Wealth (Social Circles and Emotion)

- *Basic description.* Rob Wealth individuals are passionate and opinionated and will have strong desires. Such individuals are very clear and are good at expressing their emotions. Additionally, they are good at socializing.

- *Positive description.* If they are positive, they will be independent, ambitious, convincing and eloquent. They have a strong presence—hence they will dominate a room easily. Furthermore, they adapt socially and are good talkers. In addition, they have the ability to help other people make money.

- *Negative description.* They will be jealous and anxious and have problems with friends, brothers and family. Furthermore, people will betray them. The negative Rob Wealth individual will have a double personality, one for inside and one for outside people. They will gamble and do bad things with money. They can easily lose everything at once.

Eating God (Knowledge and Intelligence)

- *Basic description.* Eating God individuals are beautiful people on the inside with lots of talent, but still they stay humble. They have a strong artistic sense and can express things clearly. Furthermore, they have a good expression of knowledge, are good writers and are very creative. It is the basic energy for prosperity and happiness. These people will have a tendency to travel, and things they do will stay strong over time.

- *Positive description.* They are humble and honest. In addition, they know how to appreciate things and are therefore always happy. They are very strong in strategy and good with metaphysical things. Moreover, they are very respectful of traditions.

- *Negative description.* The negative aspect of Eating God individuals is that they are consuming all the time. They are idealists and perfectionists. They will never listen to people and are always frustrated with their career because they are always disappointed with things. They dream of a better life and a better world. Sometimes they cannot do what they want because it is only in their mind and not in reality. This can give them the feeling of being blocked. If the individual is a woman, she will have a problem with children or a difficult relationship.

Hurting Officer (Knowledge and Intelligence)

- *Basic description.* Hurting Officer individuals will be very good at their work and career but not at relationships. They like celebrity and fame. They will fool around but will do good things; however, they want people to see that they are doing this. Moreover, they will be very creative, spontaneous and visibly talented, and can even be geniuses.

- *Positive description.* They know everything by thinking; they have no intuition but are quick to understand and learn things. Hurting Officer individuals are innovators, very ambitious and combative, and like money. They want to be different but, on the other hand, they like a good appearance and to present themselves well.

- *Negative description.* They will go against the law and they will not care if they do something bad to get things done. Other negative aspects are stubbornness, having a superiority complex and being egotistical. They will do too many things and have difficulty developing basic qualities. Since they will also repeat their mistakes, they will have chronic diseases. In addition, they will have difficulties with people they have to work with.

Indirect Wealth (Action, Prosperity and Responsibility)

- *Basic description.* Indirect Wealth individuals will look for instant and secondary money. Furthermore, they will play and gamble but will also have a talent for investing. They will enjoy action.

- *Positive description.* If they are positive they will be very competent and adult but also like to take risks. They are good gamblers and also have the ability to find good opportunities.

- *Negative description.* The negative aspect will be instability and being too fast, with no respect for money. Indirect Wealth individuals will be liars and will say yes even if they mean no. Furthermore, they can easily be cheated themselves. If it is a man, they will have a conflict with their father.

Direct Wealth (Action, Prosperity and Responsibility)

- *Basic description.* Those who are Direct Wealth like things that are clear and balanced and do not like to be in the spotlight. The balance makes them also want things to feel good. As for money, it needs to be regular and simple. Furthermore, they are classic and like nice furniture.

- *Positive description.* They will work hard and save money. Other positive aspects will be responsibility, but they also like things to be the way that they should be.

- *Negative description.* They like to save money but, with the negative, they can become mean and will even have little money. Action will be a problem for them, and as a result they will be careful in doing things, performing, and will never try to do more. They will think before doing anything. If it is a man, they will have problems with women, their wife or marriage.

Seven Killings (Power, Discipline and Organization)

- *Basic description.* These people are authoritative and very energetic. They like to use their power. Furthermore, they are tough people and like this to do with the military and weaponry. They think things should be done the way they are supposed to be done. However, at the same time, they do not like normality, and they even like to be a little bit different.

- *Positive description.* Seven Killings individuals are altruistic, persevering and ambitious. They are always alert and looking, never asleep. In addition, they do not like people who do not look straight or are not clear in character. Action and adrenaline are what they like, and they are always up for a challenge. They are charismatic leaders and will use their power in a good way.

- *Negative description.* These people will either charge into battle or be scared of everything. Seven Killings individuals will have bad habits and will not understand why people do not like the same things as them. Moreover, they are competitive, unstable, vengeful, destructive and defensive. Their energy is very reactive and they can easily lose control in life.

Direct Officer (Power, Discipline and Organization)

- *Basic description.* Direct Officer individuals are loyal, rational, moralistic and responsible and have a critical eye about themselves. These people are traditional, have values and defend the law.

- *Positive description.* They are objective, and respect rules and society. Furthermore, they respect other people's opinions. Direct Officer individuals are very calm and tranquil people. We can depend on them and they work very well with people. They will do what they are taught and can talk under pressure. In addition, they can only use good money or money that they have deserved.

- *Negative description.* These people will have an inferiority complex and be a little soft and too nice. They are not good leaders and will always follow, even to the point of going against the law.

Other negative aspects of Direct Officer individuals are difficulty in planning and acting because of rules, and they will have no initiative or creativity. Moreover, they will not be recognized by society and can only do things they are taught. If the individual is a woman, she will have problems with people she lives with.

Indirect Resource (Knowledge, Wisdom and Intuition)

- *Basic description.* Indirect Resource individuals will experience weird things such as magic and ghosts. Luck and accidents will affect them, as will unexplained events in life. They will like esotericism and spirits, but these will most likely live in their mind. They will have very strong dreams.

- *Positive description.* They will be strong, and clear in their thinking. They will have a talent for learning. Furthermore, they will have and be spiritual guides. At the same time, they will feel things and use this feeling to know about things. In addition, they will look for comfort and money and won't bother with basic needs. Other qualities they have are calmness and the ability to adapt.

- *Negative description.* They will take short cuts but cannot finish things. The negative Indirect Resource individual will be eccentric, weird, a loner and superstitious. Moreover, there is a tendency to be suicidal if things do not go their

way. A woman will have problems with her
mother, or her mother will be sick.

Direct Resource (Knowledge, Wisdom and Intuition)

- *Basic description.* Those who are Direct Resource
  individuals have a very precise image of
  themselves. They will seek and get a good
  reputation. They will have a tendency to go
  towards spirituality. They will be nice, calm,
  patient, responsible and polite. Moreover, they
  will normally move slowly and will look for
  knowledge in order to be cultivated and wise.

- *Positive description.* Cultivation and education are
  key words for Direct Resource individuals. They
  will have a good head and be generous. They
  love everything that increases the quality of the
  world and will want to help people. In addition,
  they will be very politically correct.

- *Negative description.* Negative aspects are that they
  will have problems learning things and even may
  be dyslexic. Negative Direct Resource individuals
  will be too satisfied with themselves and abuse
  their power. They will be lazy, depend on others,
  and will always try to look for comfort and
  luxury. Furthermore, they will do bad things to
  get money and will be bad in business. They have
  a tendency to be forced to take on many jobs.

The ten gods and the Day Master

Use the strength of the Day Master in relationship with the season to see the strength of the other elements, which in combination with the five factors gives us the relationship of the ten gods.

The ten gods will be more dependent on where you are age-wise in the pillar. For example, a child will be more affected by the Year pillar, because they are at the start of their lives. The ten gods each represent a different Day Master, and this is in relationship with the 'active' pillar representing your stage of life.

The relationships in the heavenly stems and earthly branches

In this section, we look at some of the relationships that are important with regard to gaining a deeper understanding of the Ba Zi. These will be the relationships between the elements of the heavenly stems and also for the earthly branches. What is important to note is that the Ba Zi is firmly set! If there is anything wrong, for example all elements are yin or there is just water present, it is very difficult to correct. This is in some ways unfair, but we need to make a big effort to change it.

Remember that in the previous sections we also looked at the Luck pillars. We can also find the relationships here with regard to the Day pillar. Hence, for a period we will have extra things affecting us. In terms of how to interpret them, these will always be considered as indirect. This will be more clearly explained below. At this point we will only look at the eight palaces and not the hidden stems.

Combinations

The combinations create an element. Again, we are looking at balance in the Ba Zi. Therefore, an extra element can balance or unbalance it. They will be considered a combination if they are in adjacent columns or separated by one column.

HEAVENLY STEMS COMBINATIONS

- Jia and Ji: earth
- Yi and Gen: metal
- Bing and Xin: water
- Ding and Ren: wood
- Wu and Gui: fire

EARTHLY BRANCHES COMBINATIONS

- Zi (Rat) and Chou (Ox): earth
- Yin (Tiger) and Hai (Pig): wood
- Mao (Rabbit) and Xu (Dog): fire
- Chen (Dragon) and You (Rooster): metal
- Shen (Monkey) and Si (Snake): water
- Wei (Goat) and Wu (Horse): fire

EARTHLY BRANCHES THREE COMBINATIONS

- Yin (Tiger), Wu (Horse) and Xu (Dog): fire
- Hai (Pig), Mao (Rabbit) and Wei (Goat): wood

- Shen (Monkey), Zi (Rat) and Chen (Dragon): water
- Si (Snake), You (Rooster) and Chou (Ox): metal

THREE ANIMALS OF THE SEASON COMBINATIONS

These combinations create a very strong element and again can be either good or bad:

- Spring: Yin Mao Chen: wood
- Summer: Si Wu Wei: fire
- Fall: Shen You Xu: metal
- Winter: Hai Zi Chou: water

Clashes

Clashes are a kind of opposing and repelling relationship. There are two kinds of clashes:

- *Direct:* Adjacent palaces (very strong).
- *Indirect:* Separated by one or two palaces (weak and subtle).

For clashes in the Luck pillars (Day pillar vs Luck pillars), we will always look at them as indirect.

EARTHLY BRANCHES CLASHES

- Zi (Rat) and Wu (Horse). This gives us worries and uneasiness. Things will trouble us and we will not be peaceful.

- Chou (Ox) and Wei (Goat). There will be obstacles and blockages. Things or people always block us.

- Shen (Monkey) and Yin (Tiger). This will bring strong emotions and will stop us from doing what we are supposed to do.

- Mao (Rabbit) and You (Rooster). A clash of these animals will be about betrayal, and people close to us will betray us. Alternatively, we will lose the trust of close friends or family.

- Chen (Dragon) and Xu (Dog). This will be about bad relationships with our children or spouse. It can also be about a shorter life span, for example an accident, or a bad habit for a time.

- Si (Snake) and Hai (Pig). Somebody will interfere with our business or personal life. People bother us and try to help us even if we do not want it. Who it is depends on which column it is in.

The harm

This relationship is about large emotions. It is what we feel inside of us. It can be emotional harm or immature emotions. Additionally, it might also be about betrayal or bad relationships with people. We will also need to look at where it is in our Ba Zi to see which relationship will be affected.

- *Indirect clash*. It is okay and can be sorted out by logic.

- *Direct clash*. The emotions are stronger than the thinking.

The clashes are:

- Zi (Rat) and Wei (Goat)
- Yin (Tiger) and Si (Snake)
- Shen (Monkey) and Hai (Pig)
- Chou (Ox) and Wu (Horse)
- Mao (Rabbit) and Chen (Dragon)
- You (Rooster) and Xu (Dog).

Ungrateful punishment

Ungrateful punishment is about not being recognized, the feeling of abandonment and being unappreciated.

The clashes are:

- Yin (Tiger) and Si (Snake)
- Si (Snake) and Shen (Monkey)
- Shen (Monkey) and Yin (Tiger).

Bullying punishment

This punishment manifests itself as a feeling within us that the world is bullying us—that the world is aggressive toward us.

The clashes are:

- Wei (Goat) and Chou (Ox)
- Chou (Ox) and Xu (Dog)
- Xu (Dog) and Wei (Goat).

Uncivilized punishment

This is about a situation that threatens us. It can be a physical threat or us being disloyal to other people. Alternatively, it can be something perceived as being unfair.

The clashes are:

- Mao (Rabbit) and Si (Snake).

Self-punishment

This comprises bad habits that we cannot stop or are very difficult to stop, such as smoking, eating, taking drugs and getting too little sleep. These are very difficult to get rid of because they are really us.

The clashes are:

- 2×Chen (Dragon)
- 2×Wu (Horse)
- 2×You (Rooster)
- 2×Hai (Pig).

Earthly branches destruction

When two specific animals appear together, they will destroy each other. As with the creation of an element, this will either balance or unbalance our Ba Zi.

The destructions are:

- Zi (Rat) and You (Rooster): yang water and yin metal
- Shen (Monkey) and Si (Snake): yang metal and yin fire

- Chen (Dragon) and Chou (Ox): yang earth and yin earth

- Wu (Horse) and Mao (Rabbit): yang fire and yin wood

- Yin (Tiger) and Hai (Pig): yang wood and yin water

- Xu (Dog) and Wei (Goat): yang earth and yin earth. This also appears in bullying punishment and they negate each other.

Three crosses

The three crosses are three exceptional combinations of four earthly branches. They are:

- *Love-success cross.* Zi (Rat), Wu (Horse), You (Rooster) and Mao (Rabbit). Such individuals will be attracted to power, celebrity, love and so on. These people will have a great capacity to attract other people (good or bad) and will be the center of attention.

- *Artistic-literature cross.* Chou (Ox), Wei (Goat), Xu (Dog) and Chen (Dragon). Such individuals will have a very strong artistic sense and will express their creativity.

- *Traveling cross.* Hai (Pig), Si (Snake), Shen (Monkey) and Yin (Tiger). Such individuals will feel at home everywhere and will move around and travel.

The void (emptiness)

The void is specific to our school and comprises the Ba Zi and heavenly systems together. We take the Jia Zi (Day pillar, Tian Gan and Di Zhi) and look it up in the table given below. The two animals that are given will determine if we have emptiness in our Ba Zi. If we have one of the animals present in our Di Zhi row, we have a single void. If we have both or one of them present twice, then we have a double void:

- *Single void.* This will be a person thinking too much and a person being upset by it. Furthermore, we will also question ourselves.

- *Double void.* This is so strong that it will completely block our Ba Zi. We need support from people and to ask people if what we do is good.

	Earthly branches											
	Yin	Mao	Chen	Si	Wu	Wei	Shen	You	Xu	Hai	Zi	Chou
Jia	Zi|Chou		Yin|Mao		Chen|Si		Wu|Wei		Shen|You		Xu|Hai	
Yi		Zi|Chou		Yin|Mao		Chen|Si		Wu|Wei		Shen|You		Xu|Hai
Bing	Xu|Hai		Zi|Chou		Yin|Mao		Chen|Si		Wu|Wei		Shen|You	
Ding		Xu|Hai		Zi|Chou		Yin|Mao		Chen|Si		Wu|Wei		Shen|You
Wu	Shen|You		Xu|Hai		Zi|Chou		Yin|Mao		Chen|Si		Wu|Wei	
Ji		Shen|You		Xu|Hai		Zi|Chou		Yin|Mao		Chen|Si		Wu|Wei
Geng	Wu|Wei		Shen|You		Xu|Hai		Zi|Chou		Yin|Mao		Chen|Si	
Xin		Wu|Wei		Shen|You		Xu|Hai		Zi|Chou		Yin|Mao		Chen|Si
Ren	Chen|Si		Wu|Wei		Shen|You		Xu|Hai		Zi|Chou		Yin|Mao	
Gui		Chen|Si		Wu|Wei		Shen|You		Xu|Hai		Zi|Chou		Yin|Mao

Heavenly stems

Good and bad pillars

In this section, we look further at different combinations but now in both the heavenly stems and earthly branches. These combinations are the strongest when they are in the same column, but can also be in adjacent palaces or on the diagonal. Also, just for simplicity, we look at the earthly branches as heavenly stems; for example, if we have Si (Snake), we look at it as yin fire. Note that in some cases it will be important to determine which element is at the top and which is at the bottom, though this will be stated clearly.

Bad pillars

The bad pillars are combinations which bring outcomes that are not good.

- Yang wood ↔ yang metal or yin wood ↔ yin metal. These people will never be satisfied because they go against themselves. They are on auto-destruct. If the combination is in the spiritual column (hour) they are not spiritual. If it is in the emotional column (month) they love to dive into deep emotions.

- Yin earth ↔ yang water. The image is that of the great flood. There will be a lot of anguish, anxiety and insecurity. Such individuals will never feel protected or safe.

- Yin earth ↔ yin water. This is the bad side of empathy. It is a sensitivity issue. Such individuals will feel that everything is so sad. There is too much emotion and they cannot digest it. Note that the primary cause of internal disease is emotions.

- Yang fire ↔ yang metal or yin metal. These people will have a very powerful ego and consequently never listen to people. If other people do not tell them exactly what they want, they will be easily upset.

- Yang fire ↔ yang water. The fire that sinks into the water. Many of these individuals were born during the 1980s. Being young, they think they can do many different things but, in actuality, they cannot do anything. If this is in their Month or Year pillar, everything they build will always be off or always wrong.

- Yin fire ↔ yin water. If these individuals are seriously into spirituality and if they have yang fire in the hour column, this takes them into non-duality. They have the capacity to accept everything and do not need to judge! On the other hand, if they are not into spirituality, the effect will be as follows:

  - *Day column:* They do not know how to choose.

  - *Emotional column:* They will have all their emotions mixed. They will not know if they are happy or sad. Furthermore, they cannot make choices and cannot be strong in their decisions.

Good pillars

Then we have the good pillars, which bring outcomes that are very good!

- Yang wood ↔ yin wood. There will be a feeling of protection and friendship. This will bring a good feeling and it gives such individuals the capacity to build things. If this is in the adjacent palaces of Day and Month, it will make them very close to their family. Additionally, they will be very close to their friends and have the possibility to build things together.

- Any wood with yin earth. This is about the capacity for development, to make something big happen and to be wealthy. If they have yin wood and yin earth in the same pillar they will have the capacity to develop a lot. For example, if the combination is in their spiritual column, they have the possibility to develop it to a very high extent. It is not the same as yang fire in the column because it is already spiritual.

- Yang earth ↔ yang water. This is a very strong combination. Such individuals will travel the world and be an explorer. They will have a lot of courage and stability. It is the pillar of possibilities! If the combination is in their Year pillar, they will always do new things and people will love them! Even with risky things it will work. It is about strength, energy and always doing new things.

- Yang fire ↔ yin water. This will give something beautiful. It is a happy connection. It is about lightness and happiness.

- Yang fire (on top) ↔ yang earth (at the bottom). The image is the mountain under the sun. It is about strong idealism.

- Yin fire (on top) ↔ yin metal (at the bottom). This is a great capacity to produce and to manifest.

- Yang metal or yang earth (on top) ↔ yang wood or yang fire (at the bottom). Yang fire and yang wood need power and space. Consequently, when they are at the bottom and blocked by something really heavy such individuals can be frustrated and maybe explode with frustration, which is not good!

- Yang wood or yang water (on top) ↔ yang fire (at the bottom). This gives frustration but such individuals will never really explode, except inside themselves. However, this will never really manifest unless they see it in their Ba Zi and do something about it. It will be a strange kind of unsatisfactory feeling.

- Some pillars are just closed. Yang metal or yin metal in a pillar will block. If a pillar is double yang or yin metal this will make a wall. If this is in such individuals' Month pillar, it will completely block who they are and what they do! It is like having a wall between pillars.

Double element

Some of the pillars are strong but they need to be put into motion, otherwise they will be dead energy. To put them into motion we need a spiritual practice.

- Yin fire. This brings stress, anguish and anxiety. Such individuals will never be able to open it by themselves! They need a tradition to do it.

- Yang fire. This can be one of the greatest pillars. If such individuals are able to channel and open it, it will explode into something great! They will be the smartest person, the best at expressing their emotions, the best at their work, and feel strong in the way they handle things. It has huge spiritual possibilities. If they do not have a spiritual practice to open it, they will only think that they are the best!

- Yang water. If this is not channeled there will be too many choices. Such individuals will not be able to decide. They want to do everything now!

- Yin water. Channeling it will bring a large capacity for empathy towards others—the capacity to link with people. On the other hand, if they do not channel it, they will have lots of sensitivity but they do not do anything.

- Yin earth. Always open. Such individuals say yes to everything! They have no discrimination.

The twelve stages of chi: introduction

The main idea in Daoism is that everything changes and is in motion. Up to this point, there has been no concept of change or motion—a rhythm. The twelve stages of chi give us this concept of rhythm. They give us information not only on the Jia Zi itself but also on the Jia Zi over time—that is, the time when it will have a strong energy and when it will be weak.

Everything that is alive, every being, has a cycle. It is born, it gets older and then it dies. Chi has this same cycle. We have these waves, these tides of chi in the day, where the chi goes up—very strong yang, then yin, and so on. What the twelve stages will give us is a more precise understanding of the Jia Zi. For example, suppose a person is yang fire (Bing), but we do not recognize this in them; however, when we examine the strength of their Jia Zi it is dead, and we see that this is the reason. Therefore, we need to know about this timing, because this timing will give us the reality behind the energy that is actually there.

With the information given by the twelve stages, we will be able not only to see the strength of the chi for our Day Master, but we will also be able to look at the strength of our Day Master for each period of our life and, in addition, at each palace with all the associations and combinations. Moreover, we will be able to do the same for each of the ten gods in our Ba Zi and see the strength of each of them compared to our Day Master. From this we can then see, for example, that for some period of our life a certain god is stronger than our Day Master. This will give us a lot more information.

We can use these twelve stages for everything, but for now we will only use them for the Day Master and the ten gods. They are universal and we will find them everywhere. The stages are:

1. Growth

2. Childhood

3. Adulthood

4. Accomplishment

5. Maturity

6. Decline

7. Ailment

8. Release

9. Dormancy

10. Completion

11. Conception

12. Birth.

Traditionally we always start with growth, but in real life the first one will be conception. Conception, and then birth, growth and so on.

Note: The translations of the twelve stages of chi can sometimes be different, so take care. Look at the numbering to make sure you have it right.

The power of the twelve stages

Each of the stages has a force of chi, which is either strong, medium or weak:

Weak	Medium	Strong
Decline	Childhood	Growth
Ailment	Dormancy	Adulthood
Release	Conception	Accomplishment
Completion	Birth	Maturity

It is, however, not always a blessing that we have a strong force, because too much strength where we do not need it may in fact be worse than having a weaker force. It might even become destructive. For example, we may have a god that is bad for us that pushes us towards bad things or even a clash. If when we look at the twelve stages this god is strong, then we have a problem.

Finding the stages

First, we will find the force of the Jia Zi. In the table on the following page we have the combinations of the Tian Gan and the Di Zhi. By finding the combinations, we find the stage of chi for the Jia Zi.

Then we can do the same for the Jia Zi and put it in relationship with a Di Zhi that can be the year, the month, the day and the hour. We will then have a very precise way to see each hour, day, month and year of the stage of chi. These relationships are given in the tables that follow the table described above.

The twelve stages	Heavenly stems									
	Yang wood	Yin wood	Yang fire	Yin fire	Yang earth	Yin earth	Yang metal	Yin metal	Yang water	Yin water
1. Growth (Chang Sheng)	pig	horse	tiger	rooster	tiger	rooster	snake	rat	monkey	rabbit
2. Childhood (Mu Yu)	rat	snake	rabbit	monkey	rabbit	monkey	horse	pig	rooster	tiger
3. Adulthood (Guan Dai)	ox	dragon	dragon	goat	dragon	goat	goat	dog	dog	ox
4. Accomplishment (Lin Guan)	tiger	rabbit	snake	horse	snake	horse	monkey	rooster	pig	rat
5. Maturity (Di Wang)	rabbit	tiger	horse	snake	horse	snake	rooster	monkey	rat	pig
6. Decline (Shuai)	dragon	ox	goat	dragon	goat	dragon	dog	goat	ox	dog
7. Ailment (Bing)	snake	rat	monkey	rabbit	monkey	rabbit	pig	horse	tiger	rooster
8. Release (Si)	horse	pig	rooster	tiger	rooster	tiger	rat	snake	rabbit	monkey
9. Dormancy (Mu)	goat	dog	dog	ox	dog	ox	ox	dragon	dragon	goat
10. Completion (Ju)	monkey	rooster	pig	rat	pig	rat	tiger	rabbit	snake	horse
11. Conception (Tai)	rooster	monkey	rat	pig	rat	pig	rabbit	tiger	horse	snake
12. Birth (Yang)	dog	goat	ox	dog	ox	dog	dragon	ox	goat	dragon

Jia Zi		Hai Pig	Zi Rat	Chou Ox	Yin Tiger	Mao Rabbit	Chen Dragon	Si Snake	Wu Horse	Wei Goat	Shen Monkey	You Rooster	Xu Dog
	Earthly branches												
	Jia|Zi	1	2	3	4	5	6	7	8	9	10	11	12
	Jia|Xu	1	2	3	4	5	6	7	8	9	10	11	12
	Jia|Shen	1	2	3	4	5	6	7	8	9	10	11	12
	Jia|Wu	1	2	3	4	5	6	7	8	9	10	11	12
	Jia|Chen	1	2	3	4	5	6	7	8	9	10	11	12
	Jia|Yin	7	1	3	4	5	6	7	8	9	10	11	12
	Yi|Chou	8	7	6	5	4	3	2	1	12	11	10	9
	Yi|Hai	8	7	6	5	4	3	2	1	12	11	10	9
	Yi|You	8	7	6	5	4	3	2	1	12	11	10	9
	Yi|Wei	8	7	6	5	4	3	2	1	12	11	10	9
	Yi|Si	1	7	6	5	4	3	2	1	12	11	10	9
	Yi|Mao	1	5	6	5	4	3	2	1	12	11	10	9

Jia Zi	Earthly branches											
	Hai Pig	Zi Rat	Chou Ox	Yin Tiger	Mao Rabbit	Chen Dragon	Si Snake	Wu Horse	Wei Goat	Shen Monkey	You Rooster	Xu Dog
Bing|Yin	10	11	12	1	2	3	4	5	6	7	8	9
Bing|Zi	10	11	12	1	2	3	4	5	6	7	8	9
Bing|Xu	10	11	12	1	2	3	4	5	6	7	8	9
Bing|Shen	10	11	12	1	2	3	4	5	6	7	8	9
Bing|Wu	8	11	12	1	2	3	4	5	6	7	8	9
Bing|Chen	8	4	12	1	2	3	4	5	6	7	8	9
Ding|Mao	11	10	9	8	7	6	5	4	3	2	1	12
Ding|Chou	11	10	9	8	7	6	5	4	3	2	1	12
Ding|Hai	11	10	9	8	7	6	5	4	3	2	1	12
Ding|You	11	10	9	8	7	6	5	4	3	2	1	12
Ding|Wei	10	2	9	8	7	6	5	4	3	2	1	12
Ding|Si	10	2	9	8	7	6	5	4	3	2	1	12

		Hai Pig	Zi Rat	Chou Ox	Yin Tiger	Mao Rabbit	Chen Dragon	Si Snake	Wu Horse	Wei Goat	Shen Monkey	You Rooster	Xu Dog
Jia Zi	Wu|Chen	10	11	12	1	2	3	4	5	6	7	8	9
	Wu|Yin	10	11	12	1	2	3	4	5	6	7	8	9
	Wu|Zi	10	11	12	1	2	3	4	5	6	7	8	9
	Wu|Xu	10	11	12	1	2	3	4	5	6	7	8	9
	Wu|Shen	11	7	12	1	2	3	4	5	6	7	8	9
	Wu|Wu	11	7	12	1	2	3	4	5	6	7	8	9
	Ji|Si	11	10	9	8	7	6	5	4	3	2	1	12
	Ji|Mao	11	10	9	8	7	6	5	4	3	2	1	12
	Ji|Chou	11	10	9	8	7	6	5	4	3	2	1	12
	Ji|Hai	11	10	9	8	7	6	5	4	3	2	1	12
	Ji|You	10	11	9	8	7	6	5	4	3	2	1	12
	Ji|Wei	10	11	9	8	7	6	5	4	3	2	1	12

Earthly branches

| | Earthly branches | | | | | | | | | | | |
	Hai Pig	Zi Rat	Chou Ox	Yin Tiger	Mao Rabbit	Chen Dragon	Si Snake	Wu Horse	Wei Goat	Shen Monkey	You Rooster	Xu Dog
Geng|Wu	7	8	9	10	11	12	1	2	3	4	5	6
Geng|Chen	7	8	9	10	11	12	1	2	3	4	5	6
Geng|Yin	7	8	9	10	11	12	1	2	3	4	5	6
Geng|Zi	7	8	9	10	11	12	1	2	3	4	5	6
Geng|Xu	11	10	9	10	11	12	1	2	3	4	5	6
Geng|Shen	11	10	9	10	11	12	1	2	3	4	5	6
Xin|Wei	2	1	12	11	10	9	8	7	6	5	4	3
Xin|Si	2	1	12	11	10	9	8	7	6	5	4	3
Xin|Mao	2	1	12	11	10	9	8	7	6	5	4	3
Xin|Chou	2	1	12	11	10	9	8	7	6	5	4	3
Xin|Hai	7	11	12	11	10	9	8	7	6	5	4	3
Xin|You	7	11	12	11	10	9	8	7	6	5	4	3

Jia Zi

Jia Zi	Earthly branches											
	Hai Pig	Zi Rat	Chou Ox	Yin Tiger	Mao Rabbit	Chen Dragon	Si Snake	Wu Horse	Wei Goat	Shen Monkey	You Rooster	Xu Dog
Ren|Shen	4	5	6	7	8	9	10	11	12	1	2	3
Ren|Wu	4	5	6	7	8	9	10	11	12	1	2	3
Ren|Chen	4	5	6	7	8	9	10	11	12	1	2	3
Ren|Yin	4	5	6	7	8	9	10	11	12	1	2	3
Ren|Zi	2	10	6	7	8	9	10	11	12	1	2	3
Ren|Xu	2	10	6	7	8	9	10	11	12	1	2	3
Gui|You	5	4	3	2	1	12	11	10	9	8	7	6
Gui|Wei	5	4	3	2	1	12	11	10	9	8	7	6
Gui|Si	5	4	3	2	1	12	11	10	9	8	7	6
Gui|Mao	5	4	3	2	1	12	11	10	9	8	7	6
Gui|Chou	4	8	3	2	1	12	11	10	9	8	7	6
Gui|Hai	4	8	3	2	1	12	11	10	9	8	7	6

An example for comparison is given below:

	Hour	Day	Month	Year
	Retirement 52+	Adulthood 35–51	Adolescence 18–34	Childhood <18
Tian Gan		X		
Di Zhi	0	X	0	0

We also have to remember that we have the hidden stems. Therefore, we have the possibility to compare these over time as well:

	Hour	Day	Month	Year
	Retirement 52+	Adulthood 35–51	Adolescence 18–34	Childhood <18
Tian Gan				
Di Zhi	0	0	0	X
Hidden stem				X

With regard to the Day Master

Again, the first thing to see is the force and state of the Day Master. By looking at the Day Master itself, plus the branch, it will give us our stage of chi. Then by relating our Day Master with the branch of the Year, Month, Day or Hour palace, it will give us the strength of our Day Master during our life.

	Hour	Day	Month	Year
	Retirement 52+	Adulthood 35–51	Adolescence 18–34	Childhood <18
Tian Gan		X		
Di Zhi	0	0	0	0

It will also give us a way to see ourselves, and the way we feel about ourselves, during the different parts of our life:

	Tian Gan	Di Zhi
Hour		My own aspiration and the relationship to my children.
Day	Day Master	The relationship between myself and partner.
Month		My personal and close family relationship.
Year		My outside and work relationship.

All this gives us additional information for our Day Master. It will be very interesting to see not only how the Day Master evolves or declines during our life but how it will also explain many other things in our Ba Zi.

With regard to the ten gods

Not only can we look at the stage of our Day Master but we can also look at it for the ten gods. For each of them we can look at their rhythm over time. As we have seen before, we can make many comparisons, which will relate to the different aspects of our lives: job, partner, children and so on.

The table below shows an example of looking at the god in the month column of the heavenly stem. This can also be used for the year and hour.

	Hour	Day	Month	Year
	Retirement 52+	Adulthood 35–51	Adolescence 18–34	Childhood <18
Tian Gan			X	
Di Zhi	0	0	0	0

Remember that we also have the ten gods in the hidden stem. An example is given in the next table:

	Hour	Day	Month	Year
	Retirement 52+	Adulthood 35–51	Adolescence 18–34	Childhood <18
Tian Gan				
Di Zhi	0	0	0	0
Hidden stem				X

We can then compare this relationship between the Day Master and the ten gods to have a complete idea of the energy given to us at different times for our Day Master and our ten gods, which is the way we will see the world.

The Day Master and the ten gods: year, month, day and hour

We cando even more with these tables. We can look at each of the Jia Zi that we compare to the Di Zhi of the hour, day, month or year.

Let us say that we want to use one of the qualities given to us by one of the ten gods. This god that we really need to use is not too strong at the time. However, by looking at the Jia Zi corresponding to the god and its branch in a calendar, we can find the best year, month, day or even hour (if we are a little obsessive) for when the expression of this god is the best time. By knowing this we can use the energy of the god much more to our advantage. On the other hand, if a god bothers us too much, we can find the time when it is weak and do the things we need to do then. This is very interesting. Furthermore, we can even do this for longer cycles. In an earlier section we talked about the Luck cycles, which were ten-year cycles. We can also apply those here.

The twelve stages of chi in detail

In this section, we give a detailed description of the twelve stages of chi. For each of them we also give a short interpretation with regard to which column they express. These are very old and traditional interpretations, which we have to interpret ourselves.

1. Growth (Strong)

Growth is about production. It is at the beginning of actual life, in between being born and not being born. Some texts say that it is after Birth, but it is not. This energy is strong, but there is a conflict because it does not know where to go. Consequently, it needs a focus, an aim. However, this energy is also very delicate.

Inside Growth, there is the idea of invention, creation, creativity, vitality and strength. It has a very strong possibility for doing things. This we need to look for. If Growth is on a useful god for us, then this will be very interesting; on the other hand, if we have Growth on something bad, then we have to take care!

Growth indicates a very strong and vibrant level of competence. We see that this gives excellence in younger years because it will really stimulate us to achieve the life we really want. If this is at the beginning of our Ba Zi, we come from a strong, smart and even rich family. Alternatively, we have a very strong and very clear resource (five aspects) where we can do many things. If we have it later, it tells us that at this time we will be able to make a lot of progress in whatever we want to do—then we can really realize what we want.

INTERPRETING GROWTH IN THE PILLARS

- *Year pillar.* If this is linked to fire it will influence the world. For a woman it can be a health problem later in life—usually after 50.

- *Month pillar.* They will not be very independent. They will have difficulties and will not be able to take advice from other people.

- *Day pillar.* They are very childish people. They will always stay very young in their heads and it will be very difficult for them to make decisions.

- *Hour pillar.* It is very difficult for such individuals to have relationships that are deep because their aspirations inside them are not very clear.

2. Childhood/Bath (Medium)

Childhood is the English translation; in Chinese it is bath, as in bathing. Bath has the image of when a baby is very young and cannot bathe themselves and hence is dependent on their mother or father for this. This is when we absorb energy that is directed at us. It is a very receptive aspect and we do not really choose other things very much. It is an absorption stage.

It will be a time where we will have romance or even just sex. There will be problems with our sexuality, being unfaithful and similar actions. It is a time when it is very dangerous for relationships. At the same time, it is a period when we are very open for relationships. Many people want to know about their love lives—we need to look at Bath because it is a time when all this sexuality is present. Furthermore, it is a very good time to meet and to attract new people.

We have this idea about sexuality but there is another thing as well, which is being very controlled or very weak in front of people. It is this image of the bath, naked child and no defense; if the parents do not hold them they will drown. It is this very helpless and very fragile thing. In addition, sometimes when we have this we have to take care because, depending on which god and which palace is active, we are a little helpless with this energy. In a relationship palace it is a sexual thing, but we are still helpless with the energy of that god. If it is related to work there is a chance that we will be manipulated or weak.

INTERPRETING BATH IN THE PILLARS

- *Year pillar.* This is very good because such individuals will get a lot of energy from their family or get good things from them. Normally they will be quite healthy for much of their life.

- *Month pillar.* They need to have support at times and make sure that they do not isolate themselves from the world.

- *Day pillar.* This is not a very strong force. They will do things but they will always miss some energy behind it. They have to find ways to get more energy.

- *Hour pillar.* Marriage will always be successful for a woman, and always unsuccessful for a man.

3. Adulthood/Formation (Strong)

This is the time when we develop ourselves. In fact, it is strict, like education—the time when we get our resources. Moreover, it is a time when we know about basic things.

For the stage of Formation it is very important that it has a resource element in its surrounding, because if it does not it means that we will be educated by people who may not have the same relationship to things or the same values as us. This means that at some point in time, now or later, it can bring trouble because we find ourselves being influenced by some values that are inside us but in fact are not actually ours. At the same time, it is a positive element—in work or association it is very good because it means that someone will help us or take us under their wing and help us do things.

INTERPRETING FORMATION IN THE PILLARS

- *Year pillar.* This means that they are strong individuals and that they have a fine family heritage. Additionally, they will keep this strongly with them.

- *Month pillar.* They will be very competitive and it will be very difficult for them to admit when they are wrong.

- *Day pillar.* They are people who will really love life, love things in life and be optimistic.

- *Hour pillar.* This will not be very good for relationships. Because they want too much, too quickly and too intensely, they will be rejected. Additionally, they will do things that other people cannot deal with.

4. Accomplishment/Starting/ Debut (Very Strong)

Debut comes after being educated and gets one ready to do things in society—a young adult trying to be independent. They may be even starting a family. It is when we are really in charge of our own destiny and in charge of our own life. This is a very strong energy because we are independent.

When we are here, it is important for all work-related matters to address questions about ourselves or for others. Promotion or being hired will be easy for us during this time, even being taken as someone better than we are. Consequently, it will be a good time to apply for a job or to sell an idea for a project. For all these types of relationships, Debut is very strong. Furthermore, we are on top, we are strong and it is a good moment to make ourselves be seen by others or to realize things, since people will see us as strong.

INTERPRETING DEBUT IN THE PILLARS

- *Year pillar.* They are strong and will be very independent.

- *Month pillar.* They will always need to work harder and a lot more than others if they want to succeed, because they are very proud and have difficulty showing what they have done if it is not perfect.

- *Day pillar.* They will not be able to work with family or people too close to them. If they do, it will not end well.

- *Hour pillar.* Their goals and aspirations will be too high. It will be difficult because they will not have a clear idea of what they can do.

5. Maturity/Prosperity (Very Strong)

Prosperity sounds good, but remember that this is Daoist thinking. It occurs when we are at the top, which means we can only go down. It is the time when we are mature but still have good vitality and we are smart with our experience. Moreover, we are still young in our minds. Again, it is an optimum point, but from here we go to the next stage, which is Decline.

When Prosperity is good, it is very good, because we have so much energy that we can do anything we want; but this is not when we especially want to look at it. When Prosperity clashes, is unfavorable or becomes a bad element for us, then we need to examine it, because a bad element with an energy of Prosperity can really result in disaster. We need to look at the cycle and time to make sure that we are prepared for whatever happens. However, it is a good moment for us to stand out or to realize things, because we will be helped and seen as somebody strong.

INTERPRETING PROSPERITY IN THE PILLARS

- *Year pillar.* They will have a very strong background and are healthy people. There are very few big health problems.

- *Month pillar.* They have a strong mind and will always need to be their own boss.

- *Day pillar.* They are independent and need to be their own boss. They are difficult to handle because they can be too strong, even bordering on arrogance.

- *Hour pillar.* They are very difficult because they are independent and too proud of what they do. This will also cause problems in relationships.

6. Decline (Weak)

We start to get older, which means we still have the Prosperity energy but it is going down. We see that some things do not go as well, and we realize that our chi is not as good. Then we have Sickness.

In Decline, and this will be the same for Sickness and Death, we have to look at negative aspects such as clashes. These negative aspects will not be strong if we have any kind of Wealth Star around, as this will neutralize it. However, if we do not, then Decline (Disease and Death also) is bad and it will bring us weakness, problems and trouble.

INTERPRETING DECLINE IN THE PILLARS

- *Year pillar.* They will be fragile and always a little sick, especially if born in the wrong season.

- *Month pillar.* They will be gentle people and will have difficulty in imposing themselves.

- *Day pillar.* They will be creative, but it is difficult for them to use their creativity for themselves. Most of the time other people will use or even steal their creations.

- *Hour pillar.* This will not always be easy for business, but for marriage it will be good. A strong relationship will always be very important for these people.

7. Ailment/Sickness/Disease (Weak)

Sickness is at the end of the energy cycle. The chi cannot defend us as well and consequently we are more fragile. We will be subject to disease and our immune system is not as good. It is just a weaker time.

See also the comments above under Decline.

INTERPRETING SICKNESS IN THE PILLARS

- *Year pillar.* Most of the time they will be sick, maybe a little or a lot, but in general they have a tendency to be sick easily.
- *Month pillar.* They will always be a little weak.
- *Day pillar.* They will worry too much, suffer from hypochondria, and lack strength.
- *Hour pillar.* They will have problems with marriage or intimate relationships, which will be recurring during their life.

8. Release/Death (Weak)

Death is when we go back to unity. It is a destruction stage. The body no longer has life but it is still there. All the subtle energy still resides there.

See also the comments above under Decline.

INTERPRETING DEATH IN THE PILLARS

- *Year pillar.* It is not a time for good health, especially if they are born in the wrong season.

- *Month pillar.* They do not listen to others, but they themselves have no good ideas either. Thus, they have a tendency to be lost.

- *Day pillar.* They will be quiet and have a very strong mind, but their thoughts will stay inside. This will be difficult because they will be always upset or frustrated.

- *Hour pillar.* A woman will marry more than once, and a man will likely be a bachelor all his life.

9. Dormancy/Tomb/Grave (Medium)

This is a time of retreat. We are in a box, under the earth. The energy is still there a little but it is slowly going back to the earth and to heaven. It is a very important time because everything is retracting into the grave. It is very important to understand that the energy is still there, but in this period it is more a conserving kind of energy. Essentially, we are keeping energy.

This idea is not bad. It is more about keeping hold of things. We can look at it as a warehouse or as a big safe where we store our energy for a little while, before it goes to the next stage of chi. Dormancy then becomes good because, if it is in combination with money, it has a great capacity to accumulate and to save. For a relationship, it is a very good period to protect it. Dormancy, because it talks about the grave, is interpreted badly most of the time, but it is actually a good thing. Of course, if it is a bad god, then it is bad because we are keeping hold of the unpleasant things.

INTERPRETING DORMANCY IN THE PILLARS

- *Year pillar.* This gives good health and a tendency to keep good health.

- *Month pillar.* Life will be easy going, with easy living. Things will be very easy.

- *Day pillar.* They will have problems with money but they will be easygoing and very optimistic in life.

- *Hour pillar.* If they get a good marriage, then they will use this marriage link to help their lives. It is therefore very important to have a good marriage.

10. Completion/Dispersion/ Disappearing/Extinction (Weak)

The extinction of life. It is when we have nothing and we go back to complete non-individuality. We are starting to go back to the Yuan Shen, and even to the Hun Dun. Life has completely disappeared from individuality and is ready to do something else, to manifest again.

In Dispersion the energy is not there, which means that the main thing at this point is that the god, element or polarity may no longer exist. If it is our Day Master it is not good, and we have to look at it very seriously, because then maybe our Day Master is not this particular Day Master.

INTERPRETING DISPERSION IN THE PILLARS

- *Year pillar.* They will do too much. They will easily overindulge in alcohol, drugs and sex, especially if they are born in the wrong season.

- *Month pillar.* They will always have periods of up and down. Things go very well and then they are nearly dead; then everything is beautiful, and afterwards they are depressed. It is like this for their whole life.

- *Day pillar.* They are abused easily and thus need to be careful.

- *Hour pillar.* They will have difficulty in trusting partners—thus it is very difficult to have a good marriage or a good relationship.

11. Conception (Medium)

In Conception, we prepare. We are doing something with intent and we are acting to do something in our new life. It is already a movement. The big thing here is that everything is possible. We have this opening—if it is on a good star, we can do almost anything we want. If it is on a bad star we still have hope, because Conception gives us all the possibilities. A bad star in Conception will be bad for us, but we do have hope.

INTERPRETING CONCEPTION IN THE PILLARS

- *Year pillar.* They will have quite good health and genes—never strong or weak, but in between.

- *Month pillar.* They will normally have a lot of illness when young but better health when grown up.

- *Day pillar.* They will be very clever—it is very good to have Conception in this pillar. They will always be a little ahead of the others.

- *Hour pillar.* They will be nonconformist and very clever but find it difficult to work hard. However, they will always find a solution.

12. Birth/Nourishing/Nutrition (Medium)

Life has been conceived. Daoist thinking says that there are ten months of being pregnant, and this encompasses all teaching before birth. Before one is born, parents get ready to teach things or become educated about raising a child. It is a pre-education time and a time for planning.

Nourishing it will bring us a type of positivity. If it is on a good star it will just tell us that it is positive; while if it is on a bad star it will just say that it is not too bad. It is this type of positive energy.

INTERPRETING NOURISHING IN THE PILLARS

- *Year pillar.* They will have quite good health during their life but not very good health. It will always be in between.

- *Month pillar.* They will have great difficulty finding themselves in their family. They will always have a feeling that it is not really their family.

- *Day pillar.* They will always want to help and do things for other people.

- *Hour pillar.* Their own life and accomplishment will be enough. Consequently, it will be difficult for them to find attraction or pleasure in meeting more people because they are satisfied in a very egocentric way.

Comments on the twelve stages of chi

The twelve stages of chi are important because they give us a better idea of each of the palaces—why they are strong or not, and how we can look at them to see their strengths or weaknesses.

Note: The descriptions above give us some idea of the stages. However, here we have given only some simple ways to teach how to use them, using just very old and traditional interpretations. In reality, they are really much bigger than this.

Conclusion

Ba Zi is a real life path; unlimited knowledge can be accessed through its study. Remember that the secret of interpretation resides in a good understanding of the basic rules: yin/yang, five elements and so on.

I hope you have enjoyed this book. I plan to do a second book where I will reveal the personalities of the sixty Jia Zi of the Day pillar. With this information, you will be able to get a good idea of someone's personality before even starting to study the chart: it is an incredible tool!

See you for the next Ba Zi book, and enjoy this ancestral knowledge!

Index